PRESCRIPTION FOR NURSES
EFFECTIVE POLITICAL ACTION

PRESCRIPTION FOR NURSES
EFFECTIVE POLITICAL ACTION

MARILYN GOLDWATER, RN
Director, Office of Federal Relations
Department of Health and Mental Hygiene
State of Maryland

with

MARY JANE LLOYD ZUSY, RN, MA
Formerly, Editor, The Maryland Nurse

Illustrated

THE C. V. MOSBY COMPANY

St. Louis • Baltimore • Philadelphia • Toronto   1990

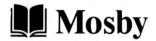 **Mosby**

Senior Editor N. Darlene Como
Developmental Editor Laurie Sparks
Project Manager Mark Spann
Production Editor Christine M. Ripperda
Design Candace F. Conner

To nurses—past, present, and future.

The C. V. Mosby Company
11830 Westline Industrial Drive, St. Louis, Missouri 63146

Library of Congress Cataloging-in-Publication Data

Goldwater, Marilyn.
  Prescription for nurses : effective political action / Marilyn
Goldwater ; with Mary Jane Lloyd Zusy.
      p.   cm.
  Includes bibliographical references.
  ISBN 0-8016-2851-2
  1. Nursing—Political aspects—United States.   I.   Zusy, Mary
Lloyd. II. Title.
  [DNLM: 1. Nursing—United States. 2. Politics—United States.
WY 16 G624p]
RT86.5.G65   1990
362.1'73'0973—dc20
DNLM/DLC
for Library of Congress   89-12912
                                                              CIP

VT/D/D   9   8   7   6   5   4   3   2   1

FOREWORD

SENATOR BARBARA A. MIKULSKI

Nurses are the front line when it comes to caring for the sick and helping the healthy stay that way. They are the professionals who provide the direct health care that so many other people just talk about. There are more than 1.2 million nurses in this country. Together they can profoundly affect our nation's health-policy decisions.

It's always been clear to me that the best ideas are the ones that come directly from the people. The best ideas about health care are the ones that come from health care professionals who work hands-on. The best policy is one that reflects the reality of nurses' lives and solves the real problems they face.

If they are to effect change, nurses must become involved in the political process at the local, state, and national levels. This how-to book takes them through that political process step-by-step. From registering to vote to under-standing how to influence the political process, from running a campaign to using the media, this book gives health care professionals a blueprint for under-standing how to become effective politically.

Think about the public debate on health care—the debate over long-term care, the ongoing problem of ensuring access to health care for all people, the constant struggle over preventing and treating disease, the increasing nursing shortage—and ask yourselves a question: will the policy that emerges from this public debate reflect my priorities and values?

You must take your values and turn them into national priorities. You must take your beliefs and make them national policy. Your ideals, your values, and your beliefs are only dreams unless you translate them into vehicles of real power.

Nurses are becoming increasingly visible and influential in shaping health policy. They are doing this by getting involved in the political process—by working with their senators and representatives, by getting appointed to local health-planning commissions, by joining their state nurses' associations, by working on those things that directly affect their lives. The more active they become, the more they increase their number, and the more clearly their voices will be heard.

This book provides nurses—and all health care professionals—with the tools to make a difference. Marilyn Goldwater has been both on the front line as a nurse and on the firing line as a member of the Maryland state legislature. She and coauthor Mary Jane Lloyd Zusy, a nurse-writer and a former editor of *The Maryland Nurse,* bring their personal experience, and with it great insight, into this work. They know what it will take to institute effective change. They have done it themselves. In *Prescription for Nurses: Effective Political Action,* they have skillfully produced a handbook on how to speed that change.

PREFACE

Politics has often been called "the art of the possible." Through it we effect change. In fact most of us engage in political activities throughout our lifetimes—many times without thinking of them as political.

For example, I often say that my first political success occurred when I was a student-nurse. In the hospital school of nursing where I studied, students assigned to the evening and night shifts for clinical experience were also required to attend daytime classes in full uniform. Many of us wanted to be able to wear street clothes to class, if we chose. I organized my fellow students to bring about this change. We petitioned the school administration and presented our case in a thoughtful and concise manner. In due course the faculty acceded to our request—it was a small political victory for all of us.

That was perhaps the beginning for me. After I graduated, Bill and I married. We had a family, and I became involved in civic efforts to improve the communities in which we lived. Because of this experience I ran for the Maryland state legislature—and won. During the 12 years I served as Delegate to the Maryland General Assembly, health policy and the advancement of professional nursing became my major interests.

During 4 of those years, I also served as a member of the American Nurses' Association's Board of Directors and chairperson of the ANA Board's Legislative Committee. Members of the committee increasingly looked at the interrelationship between politics and legislation on one hand and nursing practice and nursing education and health policy on the other hand.

In my present capacity (since 1987) as Director of the Office of Federal Relations in the Maryland State Department of Health and Mental Hygiene, I have observed the relationships between federal and state initiatives firsthand.

All these experiences have strengthened my belief that nurses must become involved in the political process at the local, state, and federal levels of government if we are to advance public health and the interests of nursing.

On the lecture circuit I talk with nurses around the country about the politics of health care. It is clear that nurses in all states are becoming increasingly visible, active, and influential in shaping health policy. On the basis of their questions and their encouragement to write a practical book on how nurses can become effective politically, I began to consider it. While all organizational work is in a sense political, my interest was to focus on government—how it works and how nurses can intervene.

During my political campaigns, Mary Jane Lloyd Zusy was a valued volunteer. Our acquaintance began when she was editor of *The Maryland Nurse*, the publication of the Maryland Nurses' Association. While she was editor of the paper, the Governor's Commission on Nursing Issues (which I chaired) published its report, making 17 recommendations to enhance recruitment and retention of nurses. Through a factual, hard-hitting series of articles written by Mary Jane, the paper played a role in influencing the decision makers to implement one recommendation: that a program of articulated nursing education within the Maryland system of higher education be developed.

I asked Mary Jane to coauthor with me the book many believed was needed. We began to meet to organize and plan. What you are about to read is the result of our work together.

This is not a textbook, but through it we hope you, our readers, will gain a better understanding of how the political system works. Through anecdotes we hope to have put flesh and bones on what otherwise might seem to be dry facts. Many of these stories are told by Maryland nurses—not because they are either unique or more exemplary than the stories politically experienced nurses in other localities might tell but because Maryland is where we live and where I have been a legislator. We hope that by sharing my political experience, we will broaden our readers' understanding of how the government actually operates. We believe that while the examples are parochial, the substance is applicable anywhere.

We will take you through the political process step-by-step—from registering to vote to holding an elective office. We will talk about networking, lobbying, risk taking, mentoring, using the media, implementing legislation, organizing a political campaign and funding it, and finally understanding the responsibilities and rewards of elective office. This is a how-to book.

While it would be meaningless to master the process without understanding the issues, exploration of issues is not the focus of this book. Intelligent stands on issues require careful study. Fortunately, there are many resources available to nurses for finding information regarding the issues that affect nursing and health care. Your professional nursing organization is one of them. We urge you to attend meetings and to read books and magazine and newspaper articles that inform you of the facts and opinions, both pro and con.

Some politicians have said, "All politics is local." We believe that. In the end politicians respond to their constituents. Voters put them in office, and they turn them out. Federal legislation is implemented at the local level. That is where citizens must see that the intent and the spirit of legislation are also implemented. This book, we hope, will motivate and inspire you to become involved in the political process in the community in which you live. Your community is the place in which you have the greatest opportunity to make the most difference.

If we as nurses are to control our professional destiny, we must understand the political process and how to use it. We hope this book will make you aware of the responsibility you bear. The book is our prescription for nurses. It would not have been possible without the many nurses who have given their support to those of us, whether elected or appointed, who have been involved in leadership positions in the shaping of health policy.

We thank our husbands, Bill Goldwater and Fred Zusy, for their support and patience during our preparation of the manuscript.

We thank Tom Lochhaas, the first person at The C.V. Mosby Company to encourage and support the idea for this book; Darlene Como, our chief editor; Linda Stagg, editorial assistant; and Laurie Sparks, our developmental editor, for their valued assistance in the development of the book; our reviewers, Karen Kelly Schutzenhofer and Roberta D. Thiry, RN, PhD, for their thoughtful reading of chapters as they were written and for their helpful comments; Judy Heffner and Sandy Sundeen for their contributions; and finally all the nurses around the country who have shared with us thoughts and experiences that will help us all to be more effective politically.

Marilyn Goldwater, RN
Mary Jane Lloyd Zusy, RN, MA

CONTENTS

Chapter 1

⫻ THE POLITICS OF HEALTH

In the course of our lifetime, vast, rapid changes in the nation's health care system have amounted to a virtual revolution. When historians chronicle these years, they will no doubt refer to the "health revolution" as readily as they refer to the Industrial Revolution. Joseph Califano, former Secretary of Health, Education, and Welfare,* once said, "The revolution in the American way of health will be as profound and turbulent as any economic and social upheaval our nation has experienced. At stake are not only billions of dollars, but who lives, who dies—and who decides." Nurses, as the major providers of health care, are—and will continue to be—profoundly affected by this revolution. The question is: Will they passively accept the changes or will they—through political involvement—play an active role in deciding how these problems are resolved?

If nursing is to take its rightful place in setting health policy, nurses must know about the issues, understand the political system, and participate in it.

Increased interest by nurses in public policy over the past 25 years has been stimulated by their realization that day-to-day professional activities are significantly influenced by government policy and programs. Many nurses have become aware that health policy directly affects how they are educated, where they practice, and how they are reimbursed.

It is in the formation of public policy that issues are raised, laws are enacted, rules and regulations developed, programs implemented, and evaluation of programs completed. It is time for nurses to be involved in the development phase of public policy. We must be proactive, not reactive.

The political issues of today are a direct result of established public policy.

The 1960s saw the development of a federal policy providing mainstream health care services for the poor and elderly. Among other programs, Medicare, the federal program that provides medical care for the elderly, and Medicaid, the state-federal partnership that provides medical care for the indigent, were passed to address the needs of these vulnerable populations. This change in health care financing gave more people access to hospital services and stimulated growth in the nursing home industry. This, along with scientific and tech-

---
*Now the Department of Health and Human Services.

nologic advances, as well as changes in patient populations, led to an increased need for more and better-prepared nurses.

To meet this need, the federal government invested more than $1.5 billion in nursing education from 1965 to 1980.

During the 1980s, federal funding for nursing education decreased significantly. Without the efforts of national nursing organizations, these funds would have been eliminated entirely. The American Nurses' Association (ANA) called upon leaders in nursing to come to Washington, D.C., and testify before congressional committees in opposition to cutting funding for nursing education. The ANA successfully stimulated a letter-writing campaign from nurses across the country to their senators and representatives in Congress. State nursing associations began to lobby state legislators for increased appropriations for programs in nursing education. In Maryland the waning federal funds, along with a growing nursing shortage, led to the creation of the Governor's Commission on Nursing Issues, which we will discuss in a later chapter.

During the 1970s the commitment to providing access to care for the elderly and poor began to weaken. As health care costs began to soar, the government looked for ways to contain them. Some states enacted legislation establishing commissions to regulate hospital rates. The federal government, through the Health Care Financing Administration headed by Carolyne K. Davis, RN, PhD, initiated studies that led to a prospective payment system as a basis for hospital charges for Medicare patients.

People who have traditionally looked to the federal government as a major source of funding for health care must now readjust their focus. Evaluation of the health care finance system is a continuous effort resulting in change and restructuring. Rising costs have made us look more closely at the related issues of access and quality of care. It is clear the system is changing.

As the crisis caused by escalating costs of health care reaches critical proportions, the public discussion surrounds three major issues—access, quality, and affordability.

Health care has become big business. Today, health care is the second-largest industry in this country, employing more than 7 million people. More than 1.2 million of these people are nurses.

A medical-industrial complex appears to be emerging. Shares of health care companies are top traders on the stock market. Competition between institutions for health care dollars and patients has made marketing their product a major activity. Institutions hire marketing experts, and a large part of many of their budgets is set aside for marketing purposes. Corporations are moving into health-promotion activities for their employees and are redesigning health care benefit packages.

In the early 1980s the cost of health care reached more than 10% of the Gross National Product (GNP).

The Health Care Financing Administration (HCFA) in a 1987 study estimated that national health expenditures will rise from $458 billion in 1986 to

$1.5 trillion by the year 2000, predicting that at that time 15% of the GNP will be spent on health care.

The health care finance system and the national health expenditures are strong forces in shaping health care policy. Other forces that shape the system as a whole and nursing as a part of that system include the health professionals, the institutions, new knowledge and technology, consumer demands, the health insurance industry, purchasers of health insurance (big business and labor are the two largest purchasers), court decisions, the media, and, last but not least, the legislative and executive branches of government at the national, state, and local levels.

Increasingly, health policy is being made by government—by elected and appointed officials who are not particularly knowledgeable about health care. They need to know that the health care system has many components with many groups of providers—and that among them nurses are the largest group. A statistic that makes legislators sit up and take notice is that 1 out of every 44 women registered to vote is a nurse.

Every legislator knows a nurse—his mother, sister, wife, cousin, aunt, or neighbor—but very few legislators understand the educational programs for nursing or the role of today's nurse. It is up to each of us individually and collectively to educate and influence the policymakers.

If we are not involved in and knowledgeable about the legislative and political processes, if we do not take the time to talk with elected officials, we have no right to expect them to know our needs or the needs of our clients.

We must also educate health consumers to the fact that our issues are their issues and that their votes count. They and their families must understand that what happens in the legislative arena directly affects what services they receive; how, where, and by whom those services are delivered; and how they are billed for the services.

The public needs to understand the different educational paths that lead to becoming a registered nurse. They need to understand the need for advanced education for nurses. They need to understand the role of the various clinical specialists. They need to know, above all, that nursing is its own art and science with its own body of knowledge that complements the art and science of medicine.

The numbers of "hyphenated" nurses—nurse-lawyers, nurse-entrepreneurs, nurse-legislators, and many others—are increasing. Such expansion is a healthy trend because the survival and growth of our profession will depend not only on those nurses who use their clinical, administrative, teaching, and research skills in their parochial environments, but also on those nurses who are breaking barriers and using their diverse skills to move into nontraditional areas for nurses. Our survival and growth will also depend on all nurses' using all their skills to make the concerns and potential of nursing heard in the forums in which decisions are being made.

We need nurses who are skilled at using the political system and the media to get our message to the public.

If we are to be effective, the public must understand the role of the nurse in today's or tomorrow's health care delivery system. If we are to influence health policy, we must be recognized as knowledgeable and respected as professionals. And we must be willing to use our potential power.

Nursing is still a profession at odds with itself. We are still plagued by divisiveness over issues such as scope of practice, autonomy, and entry into practice. In order to move ahead, it is time to end destructive divisiveness. Every nurse must understand that what helps the profession helps each of us. We must support each other. Benjamin Franklin said it so well: "We must all hang together, or assuredly we shall all hang separately."

Nursing needs women and men who are role breakers and risk takers—those with vision who work in both private and public arenas to effect positive change. They are needed at every level of nursing—local, state, and national—to articulate our strengths and accomplishments to the public.

Not everyone wants to buck the system or lead the pack. Temperament, life-styles, and family demands all influence individuals when they decide when and how much they will become involved. But, at the very least, every one of us can encourage and support those who do question and are willing to fight for needed changes. We all benefit from changes that result from their risk-taking. We must also increase the mentorship and peer support in nursing if we are to develop future leaders. We can make a difference, but our voices must be heard. Only by working together can we achieve our goals.

The future will bring even greater changes in nursing and the health care delivery system. There are exciting challenges and opportunities waiting for us, if we are prepared to accept them. If nursing is to adapt and meet the challenges, we must be the ones to reshape and redirect our profession. That is one prescription we must write ourselves.

Many people have said nursing will survive because the health care system needs nurses. The broader question is—in what shape will the nursing profession survive? Will we achieve true professional status? Will we be recognized in our new, nontraditional roles, such as nurse-entrepreneur? Will we survive in a corporate medical-industrial complex?

Nursing and the issues that surround it as a profession—scope of practice, reimbursement, image, advanced practice, and the effects of legislation and regulation—are a major focus of health care policy. Many circumstances have joined to make that so, not the least of which is the increasingly wide and obvious discrepancy between the importance and sensitivity of the work nurses do and the level of reward—economic and professional—they can expect for that work.

The most powerful reason the nursing shortage assumes urgency is obvious. We are of indispensable importance to patient care, regardless of setting or situation. When we aren't there in sufficient numbers and with appropriate skills to ensure quality care, the public is concerned and the news media take notice.

What happens to us is up to us. Becoming informed and involved—as nurses and as citizens—is crucial. Nurses in all practice settings must be knowledgeable of and active in the political process because it is this process that drives the health care delivery system. We must take our rightful place as players in the arena in which decisions are made, whether it be the U.S. Congress, state legislatures, local government, our professional associations, or the work place.

We must organize and educate ourselves, but we must go beyond our profession to the consumers (our patients), as well as other health practitioners, health planners, and administrators. Promoting itself may not come easily to a profession whose image and tradition is one of self-effacing, quiet competence in a strictly supporting role. We can maintain our competence and quality care-giving skills as we change our image and make our voices heard as both professionals and citizens. Whether or not we like it, whether or not we choose it, we are already involved in the political process. To fail to exercise the right to vote is a political act. Failure to speak up is a political act. We must not by default fail to achieve appropriate influence. Political involvement and action are keys to our future.

Chapter 2

FROM FLORENCE NIGHTINGALE TO TODAY'S POLITICAL NURSE

Trend-setting nurses from Florence Nightingale's time to our own have been effective politicians. While comparatively few have entered the political arena as candidates, many leaders in nursing have recognized a need to reform existing conditions and have organized people to work for change.

Let us focus briefly on the example set by a few of those nurses who have used their political skills to make a difference, as well as on the reasons why they have been effective and why nursing leaders have increasingly looked to legislation as a means to achieve both professional and public health care goals.

FLORENCE NIGHTINGALE: THE CONSUMMATE POLITICAL NURSE

When looking for a model of political effectiveness, we need look no further than the life story and writings of Florence Nightingale. She not only founded modern nursing but also was a world-renowned expert on sanitation, hospital reform, and the health needs of both the native people and the British army in colonial India.

Most of us know her story. She was born into an influential English family on May 12, 1820, and exhibited an early interest in service to others, care of the sick, and hospital reform. Hospitals in the mid-1800s were dirty, unsanitary, poorly ventilated warehouses of the sick and dying. Caretakers in most cases came from the dregs of society. They were untrained women, often lacking in moral character.

In an era when women's horizons were circumscribed by rigid convention, Nightingale's father was determined that his daughters get the best possible education. Under his mentorship, Nightingale acquired a stronger academic background than that of most men during her time. She was a diligent student

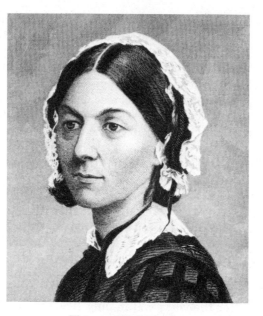

Florence Nightingale.

and was well schooled in languages, literature, philosophy, history, science, politics, and higher mathematics. Her mother rounded out her education by involving her in the everyday management of the family's two large households.

Defying the conventions of both her time and her class, Nightingale obtained what rudimentary nurses' training was available, and then essentially created professional nursing according to her own image. But it must be noted, she did so on the basis of her previous education, which was both broad and practical.

Nightingale's early efforts at hospital management were successful, but the outbreak of the Crimean War set the stage for a real demonstration of Nightingale's extraordinary abilities.

In 1854 Great Britain, France, Sardinia, and Turkey went to war with Russia to prevent that country from gaining an outlet from the Black Sea to the Mediterranean through the Turkish straits at Constantinople. Reporting from the field, a *London Times* war correspondent, William Howard Russell, wrote of incompetence, ill-preparedness, corruption, and the shocking neglect of the British wounded. He provided statistics showing that the number of soldiers who died from disease was four times the combined number of soldiers who were killed in battle or whose deaths could be directly attributed to their wounds.

Once public awareness of the desperate conditions rose, Nightingale was a natural choice to organize nursing care at the front.

Sir Sidney Herbert, British Secretary of War, appointed Nightingale Superintendent of the Female Nursing Establishment of the English General Hospitals in Turkey. He promised complete support with sufficient supplies, personnel, and medicine. Her position was strengthened by the fact that the secretary and his wife were personal friends of the Nightingale family.

Most of us know the story of Nightingale's arrival in Scutari, where a makeshift hospital had been set up. We know of her tireless efforts to organize care for the wounded against what seemed to be insurmountable obstacles. What is sometimes overlooked in these stories of the "lady with the lamp" is that she not only managed patient care but also kept records, analyzed the significance of the information she collected, and used it to strengthen reports she sent back to London. Nightingale demonstrated that the death rate at Scutari had fallen from 42% when she arrived in February 1855 to 2% 4 months later.[1]

Nightingale's remarkable work, reported in the press and in letters from the men at the front, sparked acclaim in England. With Nightingale still in the Crimea, friends and admirers conceived the idea of establishing a fund to finance a school, created by Nightingale, for training nurses. In spite of Nightingale's misgivings, the committee moved forward—with the support of the press—to collect money for the Nightingale Fund from people in all segments of society.

Four months after the war's end in July 1856, Nightingale, weakened by Crimean fever, returned to England to a public outpouring of gratitude. Financed by the fund, the Nightingale Training School of Nurses opened its doors in 1860 at St. Thomas Hospital. Nightingale had organized the first financially independent educational institution for nurses. The school became a model for others, and her *Notes on Nursing: What It Is and What It Is Not,* published in 1860, became a reference for people all over the world interested in establishing formal education for nurses.

Even while organizing the school, Nightingale was determined to bring reform to British military hospitals and to the unhealthy conditions experienced by the 70,000 British troops serving in India. In both cases she gathered information, organized it, many times illustrated it with diagrams, and presented her positions forcefully in writing and in person. Her efforts were rewarded by substantial improvements in the health and sanitary conditions of the army at home and abroad.

Nightingale continued her interest and involvement in dozens of far-reaching reforms throughout her long life. In her later years, broken by the strain of her work to organize the care of the wounded during the Crimean War, she was a semi-invalid. Confined to her room for much of the time, she counseled ministers, heads of government, reformers, and politicians. The fact that these people came to her is a tribute to her stature during her time.

Why Was She So Effective?

First, Nightingale possessed extraordinary personal qualities: intelligence, organizational ability, self-confidence, persistence, and a passion for hard work. She had visions of how things should be, and she directed her energy toward making her visions reality.

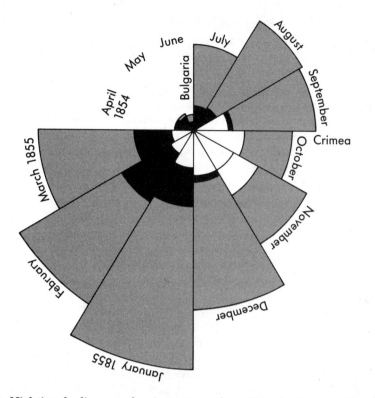

FIG. 2-1. Nightingale diagram showing extent of needless deaths in British military hospitals (1854-55). Area of wedge is proportional to statistic represented. Gray wedges, deaths from preventable diseases; white, deaths from wounds; black, deaths from all other causes. (Reprinted with permission of Tom Pantages.)

She brought to her life's work a remarkable education both theoretical and practical.

Because of her position in society, Nightingale had powerful friends who recognized her abilities and supported her endeavors. Queen Victoria was among her admirers. Nightingale was personally acquainted with every prime minister of her time. And when she went to the Crimea, the secretary of war gave her the authority to do what he had asked her to do.

The press was Nightingale's ally. Russell's reports from the field dramatized the need for nursing care for wounded British soldiers. Stories telegraphed from the front arrived in London within a day or two of their transmission. A comparison may be drawn between the speed with which news was transmitted from the Crimea and the effect it had on the British public's awareness, and the effect almost instantaneous television coverage of the Vietnam War had on the American public more than 100 years later.

The *Times* and other publications promoted the Nightingale Fund and publicized Nightingale's many calls for reform.

Nightingale was a persuasive person. Throughout her lifetime influential people came to her for advice on matters involving both nursing and public health. She was a voluminous writer and authored papers, treatises, and short books. At the front she had demonstrated her mastery of statistical analysis by documenting death rates and relating them to improvements in both care and the physical environment. Before making a proposal, she gathered data and analyzed it. Her proposals were clear and often illustrated with diagrams (see Fig. 2-1). Her writings are as understandable today as they were more than 100 years ago.

All of the nursing leaders who have followed Nightingale have had many of her qualities.

CARE OF THE SICK DURING THE AMERICAN CIVIL WAR AND ITS EFFECT ON NURSING'S FUTURE

In the United States during roughly the same period as the Crimean War, the outbreak of the Civil War (1861-1865) increased the public's awareness of the need for trained nurses. As in the Crimea, hospitals were primitive, conditions unsanitary, and relief unorganized. President Abraham Lincoln lent his support when some 600 sisters from religious orders volunteered to care for the wounded on the battlefields and in hospitals, their own and the Army's. In addition, from 2,000 to 10,000 others (depending on the source) volunteered for nursing and hospital administration. Some of these people were Dorothea Lynde Dix, Clara Barton, Louisa May Alcott, Mary Ann "Mother" Bickerdyke, and Walt Whitman.

While the war dramatized the need for trained nurses, the involvement of women from socially prominent families during that period enhanced the image of nursing and made it acceptable to the public.

In 1873 three nursing schools opened: Bellevue Training School in New York City, the Connecticut Training School in New Haven, and the Boston Training School (later named the Massachusetts General Hospital Training School for Nurses). These schools opened as independent programs separate from the hospitals with which they were associated but soon were absorbed by the hospitals because of a lack of endowment and the recognition by hospital administrators that the schools provided an inexpensive labor supply. The early 1900s saw the establishment of some 700 new schools. The purpose of the schools from the hospital point of view was service, not education. The lack of standardization of education, and of entrance and graduation requirements, became an increasing concern of nursing leaders.[2]

At the turn of the century two American nursing pioneers, Lillian D. Wald (1867-1940) and Lavinia Lloyd Dock (1858-1956), looked to legislation to solve problems they believed to be beyond the scope of the individual. Each proved her skills in the public political arena.

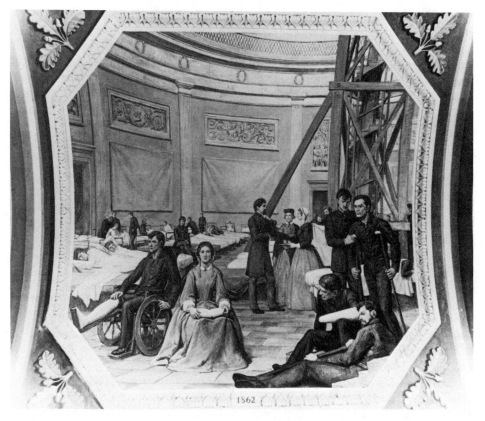

Civil War wounded are cared for in the Capitol Building. (Photo courtesy of the National Library of Medicine, Bethesda, Md.)

LILLIAN WALD: NURSE WHO SOUGHT SOCIAL REFORM THROUGH LEGISLATION

Lillian Wald was a wealthy young woman who like Nightingale took a path different from that of most young women in her social class. Following education in a private school for girls, she entered the New York Hospital School of Nursing and graduated in 1891. Within a year, however, she entered the Women's Medical College of New York.

As part of her medical school training Wald was assigned to instruct immigrant mothers on New York's lower East side in the care of the sick. This instruction became a pivotal experience in her career. Her exposure to the plight of these newcomers crowded into unsanitary tenements convinced her that the appalling social and environmental conditions in slums contributed to high death and morbidity rates in those neighborhoods. And she was determined to change them.

Wald left medical school and with her friend Mary Brewster, also a nurse, persuaded influential friends to acquire a house in the neighborhood in which they intended to work. There they established the Henry Street Settlement House, devoted to providing both care for the sick poor and the education and social services needed for them to improve their situation. The center, which later became the Henry Street Visiting Nurse Service, opened in 1893. It was the first American institution of its kind conceived and administered by a trained nurse.

The project received national attention, partly through two books authored by Wald herself: *The House on Henry Street* (1915) and *Windows on Henry Street* (1934).

The Henry Street Settlement was the beginning of organized nursing services that had a purpose beyond just care of the sick. Wald's interest was in the improvement of public health, and as time went on she broadened her original conception of community nursing. She is credited with founding all three of the major subdisciplines of community nursing—public health, rural, and school nursing.

In 1903 she demonstrated conclusively that by having nurses in the New York public schools children's absences could be dramatically reduced. Children sent home from school for health reasons in September 1902 numbered 10,567. A year later with nurses present in the schools the number of exclusions dropped to 1,101. Nurses could take care of many of the minor problems for which children previously had been sent home.[3]

Wald believed that nurses working in the community needed additional education, so she assisted Mary Adelaide Nutting in expanding course work at Teachers' College, Columbia University in New York City with fieldwork at the Henry Street Settlement.

From her "window" on Henry Street, Wald became a champion of the urban poor. She served on public commissions and investigated unemployment, cases of dispossessed tenants, children out of school because of physical defects, and working conditions among construction workers, women, and children. She enlisted the help of politicians, government officials, and philanthropists to address these problems. "I was in politics," she wrote.[4]

Repeatedly Wald looked to legislative solutions to social and health problems. She helped establish a Child Labor Committee to fight the exploitation of children by people who found them a cheap source of labor. She worked for the establishment of child-labor laws and is credited with being instrumental in the establishment of the United States Children's Bureau, the agency founded by Congress in 1912 to investigate and report on the welfare of children and to administer federal grants-in-aid to the states for maternal-child health, crippled children's services, and other child welfare programs.

She worked for improved housing in tenement districts and supported enactment of pure-food laws, education for the mentally handicapped, and passage of enlightened immigration laws.

Throughout her career, Wald exhibited vision, fearlessness, leadership, persuasiveness, and a refined sense of democracy.

LAVINIA DOCK: A SUFFRAGETTE WHO SOUGHT LICENSURE FOR THE CONTROL OF NURSING PRACTICE

During much of the same time, Wald's friend Lavinia Dock was waging two public campaigns, one for the vote for women and the second for legislation to control nursing practice.

Dock was a prolific writer and perhaps is best remembered for her contributions to nursing literature, but she was also a political activist throughout her career. She too had grown up in a well-to-do family that valued education for its daughters. Dock graduated from the Bellevue Training School for Nurses in 1886. She wrote her first book, *Materia Medica for Nurses,* while serving as a night supervisor at Bellevue Hospital.

Dock was among the early feminists, the growing number of women who believed that the way to achieve equality with men was through attainment of the right to vote. Dock was a dedicated suffragette and engaged enthusiastically in protests, marches, speeches, parades, and demonstrations. Passage of the Nineteenth Amendment to the U.S. Constitution in 1920, the amendment that gave women the right to vote, was also a milestone for nursing.

Dock often cautioned about male domination of nursing by physicians and hospital administrators. She believed that nurses should control nursing and that they must organize to achieve professional goals. First among those goals was licensure to control nursing practice. It would protect the public from untrained women who called themselves nurses and establish standards for nursing education. She believed that nursing organizations should spearhead the drive. With Isabel Hampton Robb and Nutting, she helped found the organizations that were to become the National League for Nursing (NLN) (1893).

NURSE LICENSURE, THE WOMEN'S MOVEMENT, AND NURSING'S GROWING INVOLVEMENT IN POLITICS

The struggle for nurse licensure was long and arduous, and the fight for enabling legislation had to be won in every state. Regulations varied. In most states, boards of nursing were established. In New York, applicants had to be graduates of training schools approved by the regents of the state university, but in some other states all that was required was the ability to pass an examination.[3] In 1903 New York, North Carolina, New Jersey, and Virginia were the first to pass licensure legislation. As is often the case, legislation passed in one state stimulates similar legislation in others. However, almost 20 years passed before every state (plus Hawaii and the District of Columbia) had licensing regulations in place.[2] The effort did much to strengthen and unite nursing. It represented organized nursing's first experience in the achievement of professional goals through legislation.

On the basis of this political experience, the ANA formed a legislative committee in 1923 and continued to speak for nursing through the Great Depression, World War II, and the Korean War. In 1940 the ANA and The National League for Nursing Education, later renamed the National League for Nursing (NLN), passed a joint resolution offering President Franklin Roosevelt "the support and strength of our organizations in any nursing activity in which we can be of service to the country." The ANA supported the passage of the bill that created the United States Cadet Nurse Corps in 1943[3] and testified at House hearings in support of the Nurse Training Act of 1964. But it was not until the early 1980s that the ANA became markedly more assertive in the legislative field.

In spite of the fairly recent entrance of men into the field, nursing remains a predominantly (97%) female profession. Therefore advances in nursing have often paralleled improvements in the status of women. The consciousness raising that occurred as a result of the women's movement in the 1970s and 1980s had a direct effect on nurses.

The National Organization for Women (NOW) was established in 1966 through the merger of two groups of women activists. One group, coming from essentially the well-educated white middle class, focused on issues such as pay equity (equal pay for equal work), comparable worth, continuation of wives' social security and pension rights after divorce or the death of a spouse, and equal employment opportunities. Members of the other group were younger and frequently single. Many had participated in the anti-war protests and civil rights movements of the 1960s. Their agenda was more controversial: they sought universal availability of abortion, equal rights for lesbians, and prosecution for rape within marriage, among other changes.[5]

While the abortion issue continued to separate individuals in the group, a new solidarity emerged. NOW became the largest and most vocal women's organization. During that period, a growing number of women became interested in political involvement. Nurses were among those who studied the issues, learned how to lobby for their points of view, chose candidates, worked in campaigns—and eventually ran for office themselves. In January 1989 JoAnn Zimmerman, RN, was Lieutenant Governor of Iowa; Kathleen Connell, RN, was Secretary of State of Rhode Island; Barbara Hafer, RN, was Auditor General of Pennsylvania; and 45 nurses sat in state legislatures (see Appendix A for list).

In this new environment for women, nurses became more sophisticated politically. They came to realize that legislation affects nurses' education and reimbursement, as well as the quality of patient care. They expected the ANA to assume a more assertive political stance. The organization's House of Delegates passed an increasing number of resolutions requiring legislative action. In response the ANA Legislative Committee, which I chaired from 1984 to 1988, was energized in 1981. By February 1988 the organization's Washington, D.C., office had been expanded from a staff that for many years had one lobbyist to one that included seven lobbyists and five political staff members. "Instead of just reacting to proposed legislation," said ANA Political Director Pat Ford Roegner, "we are now involved in writing it."

In 1976 the ANA established a political-action committee (PAC), which made its first campaign contributions in 1978. Originally named Nurses-Coalition for Action in Politics (N-CAP), it was later renamed ANA-PAC for easier identification. (We will talk more about the PACs in Chapter 8.)

Politicians began to value having nurses on their campaign and administrative staffs. (In November 1987 ten nurses held positions on the Capitol Hill staffs of U.S. senators.[6]) Some elected officials asked nurses to join their policy-making inner circles. Some pushed for nurses' appointments to top positions in government agencies.

CAROLYNE K. DAVIS, RN, PhD: FOURTH ADMINISTRATOR OF THE HEALTH CARE FINANCING ADMINISTRATION

In this climate of growing respect for nurses in politics, Carolyne K. Davis, RN, PhD, was appointed to a top health policy-making position in the federal government in February 1981. She was the first woman to hold the position and the fourth administrator of the Health Care Financing Administration (HCFA), U.S. Department of Health and Human Services.

During the four years Davis held the position, she was responsible for Medicare and Medicaid programs, which finance health care services for 54 million poor, elderly, and disabled people. Expenditures on their behalf totaled nearly $100 billion in fiscal year 1985, making HCFA's budget the third-largest agency budget in the federal government at that time.

During Davis's tenure the prospective payment system using diagnosis related groups (DRGs) as a basis for hospital reimbursement under Medicare was implemented. A waiver program to permit greater flexibility to the states in delivering home- and community-based health care services was developed. A Peer Review Organization program to monitor utilization and quality of care was initiated. A prospective payment system for reimbursement of health maintenance organizations (HMOs) under Medicare was implemented, and rules for coverage and reimbursement of ambulatory facilities as a cost-effective alternative to inpatient hospital services were developed. These were significant efforts toward controlling rising health care costs while at the same time attempting to safeguard the quality of health care for Medicare and Medicaid recipients.

Davis came to the HCFA position with an excellent background of nursing experience as a clinician, educator/administrator, and writer. She had been Associate Vice-President for Academic Affairs at the University of Michigan, at the same time chairing the university hospital's cost containment committee. Prior to that, she had been Dean of the University of Michigan School of Nursing and had chaired the baccalaureate nursing program at Syracuse University.

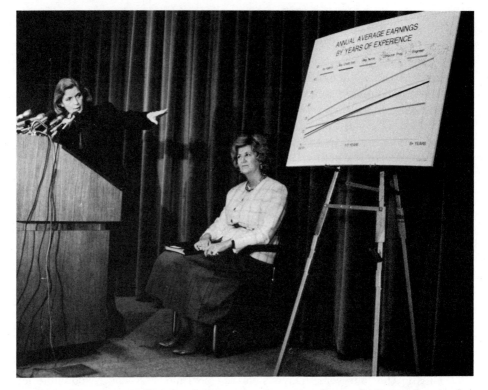

Carolyne Davis, RN, PhD (left), chairwoman of a national commission on the nursing shortage, and Lillian Gibbons, executive director, explain panel findings. (From *The Washington Times,* December 13, 1988.)

Throughout her career she has published articles and papers dealing with a wide variety of issues facing the health care system. She credits her background at the bedside as the source of her practical knowledge of how hospitals work.

But her appointment to the high-ranking position in the HCFA came as a direct result of her involvement in Michigan state politics. When Davis was administrator of the University of Michigan Health Sciences Department, Congress threatened to cut off capitation funds for nursing education nationwide. Davis and others believed that nurses should do something about it. With the help of Michigan Congressman Carl D. Pursell they organized an effort to lobby Congress directly for the restoration of the funds. Davis describes the successful effort:

> We started working with the congressman. We planned a three-day marathon campaign in the nation's capital. Sixty students and 12 university faculty members, including myself, along with some faculty and students from other institutions, boarded buses for Washington, D.C. Before leaving Ann Arbor, the congressman had helped us devise a strategy. We knew whom we wished to see and

what we planned to do. With his help we were successful. The nursing-education funds were restored.

Five or six months later it was our turn to return the favor. Congressman Pursell had never carried Washtenau County. In that county there were two hospitals. I believed the nurses employed there could be attracted to his candidacy on nursing issues and that he deserved nursing's support. Through the state board of nurse examiners, I was able to obtain for him a list of the names and addresses of the 4,104 nurses in his district.

Our next problem was how to get the nurses involved. Candidates need more than money. They need help—that is, people to stuff envelopes, fold campaign material, check lists, make phone calls, and be involved in the hundreds of activities that go into a political campaign. We posted a sign-up sheet at the school of nursing.

When volunteers were needed to pass out leaflets at a football game, nurses did it. They staffed his office the last week of the campaign. Congressman Pursell won reelection, and nurses were credited with having made a real contribution to the win.

Having become thus involved in Michigan politics, I was included in the behind-the-scenes strategy of the next presidential campaign. I found that I was good at political strategy development, and understanding it was a great advantage to me when I came to Washington. I understood the art of compromise and how to get things done.

It was Congressman Pursell who pushed my appointment to the HCFA position with newly elected president Ronald Reagan. The contacts I had made working in grass-roots campaigns in Michigan were invaluable to me in Washington. Cultivating friendships and utilizing contacts with influential people is an essential element of effectiveness in politics.[7]

More recently Davis has received national attention as chairperson of the Secretary's Commission on Nursing for the U.S. Department of Health and Human Services. In 1988 the commission studied the causes of the nursing shortage and made widely publicized recommendations designed to address these problems.

SHEILA BURKE, RN: INFLUENTIAL STAFFER FOR SENATOR ROBERT DOLE

Sheila Burke, RN, MPA, FAAN, has achieved increasing influence on Capitol Hill through her staff positions with Senator Robert Dole (R-Kan). She became chief of staff for the office of the Republican leader of the U.S. Senate in 1986. In this position Burke's responsibilities extended to the party's leadership in the Senate—a broader role than she previously had held as chief of staff for Dole's Senate office.

How did Burke achieve such an important position? "It started," she says, "with my involvement in student government at the University of San Francisco School of Nursing." Through that experience she became president of the National Student Nurses' Association (NSNA), kept her ties to the NSNA after graduation, and, after a year's experience as a hospital staff nurse, became NSNA Director of Program and Field Services in 1974.

This position brought Burke national exposure, contacts in Washington,

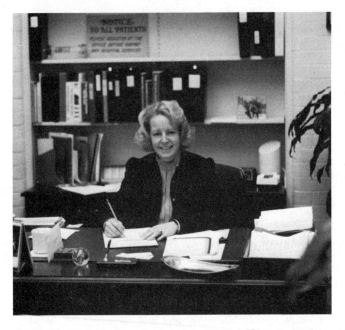

Sheila Burke, RN, MPA, FAAN, at her desk in her Capitol Hill office. (From Nursing and Health [6(5):244. 1985].)

D.C., and a growing awareness of the importance of nurses' becoming involved in the development of health policy. "I could see that there is a direct relationship between politics and how we pay for things," she says. "Since health services must be paid for, the politics of how this is done is a specific interest for nursing. Health policy is driven by the financing mechanism."

In 1977 Burke became a legislative assistant to Senator Dole. At that time she worked on the preparation of legislative proposals and amendments on matters regarding health, welfare, social security, and women's rights. Since then she has become more influential on matters of health policy. As Senator Dole's career advanced, Burke's kept pace. In 1982, she became deputy staff director of the U.S. Senate Committee on Finance, of which Senator Dole was a member. She was the staff's chief contact on such programs as Social Security, disability insurance, Medicare, Medicaid, maternal and child health, and peer review organizations.

Burke urges nurses to become involved in politics. "Nurses should approach it as a challenge," she says. "It takes time and commitment." She advises, "Begin at the grass-roots level, find out the issues, and then contribute time to a campaign for a candidate whom you think will best represent you."

Good communication skills are most important for success in the political arena in Burke's opinion. The ability to identify critical issues, translate them into language that is understandable to one's audience, and articulate the pros and cons of an issue in a concise manner are vital for effectiveness, Burke believes.[8]

HAZEL JOHNSON-BROWN, RN, PhD: FIRST BLACK WOMAN GENERAL IN THE MILITARY SERVICES

Hazel W. Johnson-Brown, RN, PhD, FAAN, used her political abilities to achieve a top position in and then to manage a large federal organization. Throughout her 28 years of service in the Army Nurse Corps (ANC) her remarkable political and organizational skills brought her promotion after promotion.

Johnson-Brown was the first black woman to reach the rank of general in the history of the military services. She was appointed brigadier general in the U.S. Army in 1979 when she became chief of the ANC. As chief she frequently testified before Congress and worked with high-ranking government officials. She knew the system when, upon retirement from the corps in 1984, she assumed the direction of the ANA's Office of Governmental Affairs in Washington, D.C., for a two-year period. There her staff worked directly with legislators and government officials to enact and implement legislation supporting nursing and ANA-endorsed health policy.

As a result of these experiences Johnson-Brown has clear ideas about the qualities that enhance political effectiveness.

"In working with people you must have a very clear understanding of the goal," she says. "Know what it is and what its impact will be." Then she puts perseverance at the top of her list of the ingredients for political success:

> People find that I am very persistent. If I don't get what I think is right the first time, I go back. If I fail, I consider why I was not successful and fix what needs fixing. I stick with positions I believe are right.
> When I campaign for something, I am willing to walk the extra mile. I always do my homework. When someone asks to see me, I try to find out something about that person and why he or she wants to talk with me. I'm also willing on some occasions to say, "I was wrong."
> Eventually people less dedicated to a course of action than I, give in.

Johnson-Brown puts negotiation and compromise skills second on her list:

> I am willing to do something to get something, as long as it doesn't compromise my integrity.
> When I campaign for the support of individuals in powerful positions, as an example, when I go to a board meeting, I know in advance who is with me and who against and why. I base my presentation on meeting the objections of those opposed.
> We have to be willing to compromise. Accept the fact that there will be opposition, and find ways to get the person opposed to come with you on some of what you want.
> Know your bottom line when you are negotiating, and try to get a compromise above it. Take a piece now, and try for another piece later. It may even be that as time goes on, you may find that it would be better to modify the position you originally took.

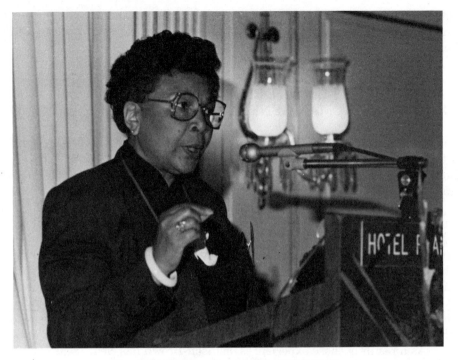

Hazel W. Johnson-Brown, RN, PhD, FAAN.

When negotiating never be afraid to lose your job because of the position you support. Fear allows opponents to deal with you in a very negative way. You must play the negotiating game, and if a group is negotiating a position do not demonstrate indecisiveness by airing disagreements in public. It is devastating to your effectiveness.

Finally Johnson-Brown believes that tact, diplomacy, the ability to sell one's ideas, and having the facts to back up one's position are essential political tools. She gives this example:

Some have wondered how we ever established the minimum requirement that those on active duty in the ANC must have graduated from an accredited nursing program and hold a baccalaureate in the science of nursing (BSN) degree. Baccalaureate education as a standard for nurses—even in the 1980s—is hotly debated by nurses and misunderstood by the public.

Chiefs of the ANC since 1955 have talked about making the BSN an entry requirement, but when the army decided in 1979 that all officers should have baccalaureate degrees, ANC leaders seized the opportunity. They began recruiting candidates with the BSN for active duty in the corps. Early efforts to make associate degree nurses warrant officers proved impractical and unsatisfactory.

In a remarkably short period of time—some 13 years—the corps was able to establish a minimum standard of nursing education for its nurses on active duty. More than 98% of those nurses now hold the BSN.

Nevertheless every chief since 1974 has had to answer questions—often from powerful people—as to why the corps maintains this standard. I explained it in terms of where we had been and where we were going—and often in terms of dollars and cents. With a common standard for entry, there is a standard for advancement. Money spent for advanced education is just that. We have statistics to show that Army staff-development courses are recognized for their excellence. They have been developed for nurses at a defined level of education and are attracting nurses from the community.[9]

SUMMING IT UP

Nurses' interest and involvement in the politics of government have closely paralleled those of other women. The campaign for women's right to vote marked the appearance of large numbers of women in public life, but it was the women's movement in the 1970s and 1980s that energized women to take their rightful places in the political arena.

After spearheading the effort for nurse licensure, the ANA continued to speak for nursing. But it was the early 1980s before the organization really expanded its interest in legislation to achieve professional and public-health goals. This expansion correlated with the changing environment for women and signaled nurses' increased interest in political activity.

What can we learn from the examples of representative nurse leaders who have made a difference? What strengths go with their kind of leadership?

Their strengths include vision and the commitment to make dreams realities; persuasiveness; tact and diplomacy; education; organizational and negotiating skills; the ability to collect and analyze information, to communicate one's positions clearly, to build networks and develop contacts, and to work with the media; an understanding of the political system; and the capacity for hard work.

Some of these talents are gifts. Others are abilities that can be developed with increased knowledge and experience. Many of them represent the skills most of us develop as nurses: the ability to communicate, observe well, process information, organize, and work with people from all socioeconomic backgrounds. In the chapters that follow, we will talk about how we as nurses can broaden these skills to make us more effective in the political arena.

REFERENCES

1. Hebert RG: Florence Nightingale: saint, reformer or rebel? Melbourne, Fla, 1981, Krieger Publishing Co Inc.
2. Donahue MP: Nursing: the finest art, St Louis, 1985, The CV Mosby Co.
3. Kalisch P and Kalisch BJ: The advance of American nursing, Boston, 1978, Little, Brown & Co, Inc.
4. Chinn PL editor: Nursing history, Advances in Nursing Science 7(2):10, 1985.
5. Archer SE and Goehner PA: Nurses: a political force, Monterey, Calif, 1982, Wadsworth Publishing Co.
6. AJN Almanac: American Journal of Nursing 87(11):1,404, 1987.

7. Davis CK: Personal communication, November 1987.
8. Burke SP: Personal communication, December 1987.
9. Johnson-Brown H: Personal communication, January 1989.

ADDITIONAL READINGS

American Nurses' Association: Nursing hall of fame, Kansas City, Mo, 1984, The Association.

Baly, ME: Florence Nightingale and the nursing legacy, Dover, NH, 1986, Croom Helm.

Bullough B, Bullough VL, and Barrett E: Nursing: a historical bibliography, New York, 1981, Garland Publishing, Inc.

Bullough VL and Bullough B: History, trends, and politics of nursing, Norwalk, Conn, 1984, Appleton-Century-Crofts.

Dolan JA, Fitzpatrick ML, and Hermann E: Nursing in society: a historical perspective, ed 15, Philadelphia, 1983, WB Saunders Co.

Kalisch PA and Kalisch BJ: The advance of American nursing, ed 2, Boston, 1986, Little, Brown & Co, Inc.

Nightingale F: How people may live and not die in India, London, 1864, Longman, Green, Longman, Roberts and Green.

Nightingale F: Introductory notes on lying-in institutions, London, 1871, Longmans, Green, and Co.

Nightingale F: Notes on nursing: what it is and what it is not, New York, 1860, Appleton & Co.

Smith FB: Florence Nightingale: reputation and power, London, 1982, Croom Helm.

Chapter 3

⫻ YOU CAN MAKE A DIFFERENCE

American women have come a long way since winning the right to vote some 70 years ago. Largely ignored or taken for granted for many years, women voters became an impressive force by the 1980s. Comprising 53% of the voting age population, women now both register and vote in greater numbers than men, and the gap between the numbers of men and women voters continues to widen.[1]

What were the forces and who were some of the people behind attainment of voting rights for women? How can we use the voting rights they won for us and participate in the political process to make a difference? And how can nurses and nursing organizations, working with other groups, use the democratic process to further health-policy goals?

THE STRUGGLE FOR WOMEN'S SUFFRAGE

Let's look briefly at how women won the vote.

Tennessee, the last state needed for ratification, passed the Nineteenth Amendment to the Constitution on August 26, 1920, thereby extending suffrage to women nationwide.

Congresswoman Jeanette Rankin of Montana—the first woman elected to Congress—introduced the constitutional amendment on January 10, 1918. When the confirmation vote came, the amendment passed by one vote more than the required two-thirds majority—dramatic testimony to the importance of just one vote.

Passage of the Nineteenth Amendment was the culmination of a hard-fought campaign, one that had been waged by a succession of a few dedicated women since the early 1800s. As early as 1792 a British woman, Mary Wollstonecraft, spoke out against all kinds of enslavement, including that of women by men, in a book titled *A Vindication of the Rights of Women*. The book became a handbook for the feminist movement throughout the world.

In the United States many feminist leaders became politically active in the antislavery movement. In fact the Women's Rights Convention held in Seneca Falls, New York, in July 1848, was called in response to an experience by two of

23

these women, Lucretia Mott and Elizabeth Cady Stanton. They—and other women—had been barred from participation in the World Anti-Slavery Convention, held in London in 1840. Women saw this as an obvious denial of their rights, and it heightened their awareness of the parallel between the unfair differences between the rights of masters and slaves and those between men and women.

More than 300 women answered the call to attend the Seneca Falls convention. The group outlined areas of women's subservience in marriage, education, franchise, property ownership, and guardianship, among others. It passed 12 resolutions calling for measures that would correct these inequities. Eleven of the proposals were readily accepted, but a 12th, introduced by Stanton and requesting the right for women to vote, was hotly debated and narrowly passed.[2] The idea of women's suffrage—even among progressive women—at that time was controversial.

During much the same period another reform movement captured the imagination and enthusiasm of many women: the growing fight for a ban on the use of alcoholic beverages, believed by many to be a serious threat to home and family. The movement became organized with the founding of the Women's Christian Temperance Union in 1874. Fortunately its leader, Frances Willard, broadened its mission to advocacy of any reform that would benefit women and children. Many women, drawn to the organization because of the temperance issue, began to see the importance of women having the right to vote.

Susan B. Anthony was one of the women who had become politically active in the temperance movement. But after meeting Stanton in 1851, she redirected her energies into the efforts to gain women's suffrage. Ultimately she became the movement's principal leader. While the movement continued, national attention in those years focused on the twin issues of slavery and states' rights and on the threat of war.

The Civil War resolved the issue of slavery. In 1868, following the war's end, the Fourteenth Amendment to the Constitution was ratified. Its purpose was to make former slaves citizens and to give them full civil rights. But it was the Fifteenth Amendment, ratified 2 years later, that made clear that those civil rights included the right to vote.

What offended Anthony and Stanton was that the vote was given to black men—but not to women, whether black or white. In protest they separated from women who had accepted the Fourteenth Amendment and formed the National Women's Suffrage Association in 1869.

In the early years backers of women's suffrage sought its mandate state by state. As nurses seeking mandatory nursing registration had found, this was no easy task. The suffrage proposal was so controversial that Anthony and Stanton concluded that to fight for it in every state legislature would be an overwhelming task. They decided that an amendment to the Constitution would solve the problem more expeditiously.

They enlisted the help of California Senator Aaron Sargent, who introduced the Anthony Amendment into the U.S. Senate. It was defeated, and for the next 40 years similar proposals were regularly reintroduced. Each time the

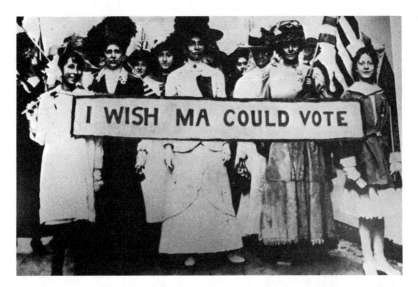

"I Wish Ma Could Vote." Painting by R. Schwartz. (Used by permission of Mr. and Mrs. Robert Kanuth.)

initiatives failed by narrower margins. At the turn of the century Wyoming and several other Western states came into the union having given women the right to vote in their state constitutions. The time for women's suffrage had come. By 1920 acceptance was broad enough nationwide for the passage and ratification of the Nineteenth Amendment. Women's right to vote became a reality.

Much more could be said about the history of the extension of enfranchisement in the United States, but that is beyond the scope of this book.

EXERCISING THE RIGHT TO VOTE: WHO DOES AND WHO DOESN'T

It is important to realize that many people have struggled through many years to attain rights of full citizenship for previously neglected segments of our population. Our most basic right is the right to vote. It is discouraging then, to find that many people do not exercise it (Fig. 3-1). Despite voter-awareness campaigns in the print and electronic media and massive registration drives, voter participation is discouragingly low. Unofficial estimates show that only 50% of people eligible to vote did so in the presidential election in 1988.[3]

Voter turnout is always greater in presidential-election years; stripped of the hoopla surrounding national contests, the turnout in state and local elections in other years frequently drops to under 25%.[4]

The Twenty-sixth Amendment, ratified on July 1, 1971, broadened enfran-

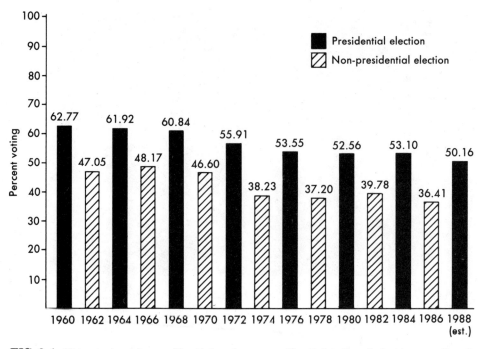

FIG. 3-1. Voter turnout in presidential and non-presidential national elections: national average of voting-age population voting for highest office. The sharp drop in voter turnout in 1972 reflects the expansion of eligibility with the enfranchisement of 18 to 20 year olds. (From Kimberling W and Flor A: Federal election statistics: Tech Rep 1, FEC Clearinghouse on Election Administration, Washington, D.C., July 1988.)

chisement by lowering the voting age from 21 to 18. In the election that followed, the percentage of eligible people who voted declined significantly. In 1968 60.6% of voters cast their ballots. In 1972, a year after the amendment's ratification, only 55.5% voted. The numbers suggest that the majority of the newly enfranchised young voters did not vote (Fig. 3-1).[5]

Surveys show that there are differences in who votes. Surveys done in 1980 showed that there was higher participation among the elderly, the better educated, whites, city people, Republicans, Northerners, and those with jobs, particularly in middle- or higher-income jobs. The same survey indicated that many fewer than half of those with only an elementary school education voted.[4]

Eleanor Smeal, a past president of NOW, points out that in terms of sheer numbers, women's voting strength is steadily growing. Since the election of Lyndon Johnson as president in 1964, more women have cast ballots in the general election than men. She notes that in 1984 a higher percentage of women than men were registered to vote and that since 1976 the percentage of registered women has increased while the percentage of registered men has decreased. She believes these figures indicate that women's influence in politics will continue to grow.[1]

As one would expect, politicians court groups of citizens who they believe will vote on election day. In recent years the elderly have become an influential voting block because they vote in large numbers. And as women have become more active politically, candidates have listened to their concerns with growing interest. Groups who can define their positions and "get out the vote" are rewarded by politicians' attention to their issues.

REGISTER TO VOTE

The U.S. Constitution originally left most regulations regarding voting up to the states. While succeeding constitutional amendments mandated that eligibility to vote be broadened nationwide, rules regarding voter registration and parties' selection of their candidates still vary from state to state and locality to locality.

In some states voting procedures were intentionally made complex. The poll tax, literacy tests, and property requirements were all regulations attached to voting that represented attempts to exclude certain groups of possible voters. These barriers have been removed, though some believe that there are still some subtle factors that work against full enfranchisement.

Voter registration has been accepted as a method of combating corruption and ensuring that each citizen casts only one vote. The actual act of registering someone to vote must be done in a non-partisan manner.

Some states make it easy for a voter to register. Several weeks before elections, registration tables are set up in shopping centers or in other highly visible public places. You can register there or request a voter registration form from your local board of elections (sometimes called the board of election supervisors) by telephone or letter. In other states you must go to the county courthouse or another designated place to register.

Most states have some sort of residency requirement; where you live determines where you will vote. Unless you vote by absentee ballot (which we will discuss a little later), you must vote in your neighborhood at the polling place designated by the election board. Once registered, you continue to vote in the same precinct unless you move. If you do move, call your board of elections to find out what you must do.

Once registered, you will receive notification of your polling place by mail. In some localities you will receive a voter registration card, which gives your name, legislative district, and polling place.

Remember that voter registration is open for a specified time before each election. If you fail to register before the primary election, you will have another opportunity to register before the general election.

If you know you will be away from home on election day—whether at school, on business, or for personal reasons—request that your board of elections mail you an application for an absentee ballot. Fill it out and mail it promptly. The ballot must be received by the board before the polls close on election day if it is to be counted.

Voter lists are trimmed every few years. The names of persons who have not voted in a specified number of years are struck from the list of eligible voters. If you are one of these persons, you must reregister to vote, even if you live in the same place.

Nurses should remind both hospitalized and homebound patients that special arrangements can be made for them to vote. Since voting regulations vary from state to state, you may want to call or write your county seat, the local offices of the League of Women Voters, or Democratic or Republican Party headquarters for information.

CHOOSING A POLITICAL PARTY

When you register to vote, you will be asked to specify a party preference, although you may register as an independent. In the United States there are two major political parties: Democratic and Republican. A few minor parties perennially put forth a limited slate of candidates, and once in a while a "third" party forms around the candidacy of a real contender who shuns both major parties, for example, Henry Wallace and the Progressive Party in 1948.

Regardless of how you intend to vote in the general election, there is great value in choosing the major party that best represents your political philosophy when you register. Many people like to think of themselves as independent voters, but in registering as such they miss the opportunity to vote in the pri-

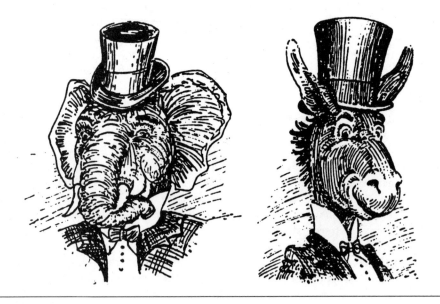

maries in most states. It is through the primaries in these states that the parties select their candidates for the general election. With the exception of states that hold open primaries, if you are a Democrat you vote in the Democratic primary, and if you are a Republican you vote in the Republican primary. As an independent you can vote in neither primary, so you lose a vital opportunity to have an influence.

In the general election, no matter what their party affiliation, people are free to vote for candidates of any party.

HOW DO PRIMARIES WORK?

Most states hold direct primaries. In these spring elections, voters go to the polls to choose between candidates in their own parties. They also may choose delegates to the party's national convention. Voters go to the polls, are identified as Democrats or Republicans, and are given an appropriate ballot.

A few states hold open primaries, in which both Democratic and Republican candidates appear on one ballot and voters can choose to vote in the primary of either party.

Some states choose presidential candidates through party caucuses or conventions. In these states, party members meet in designated places around the state to campaign for their candidates and to cast their votes. In 1988 caucuses were held in 18 states.* The parties decide how their candidates are selected, and they can change their systems periodically. As you can see, once more you need to learn about the specifics of how the system works in your community. The League of Women Voters, the office of your political party, or your local board of elections can give you that information.

VOTER REGISTRATION DRIVES:
REASONS FOR THEIR ORGANIZATION AND
AN EXAMPLE OF A NURSE-ORGANIZED DRIVE

Boards of elections, the League of Women Voters, and other non-partisan groups interested in increasing voter participation mount voter registration drives before elections. In recent years, however, both political parties and other interested groups—including nurses—have promoted voter registration in an effort to activate certain groups of people who may not have participated regularly in the election process. While registration does not include any commitment to vote in any way, activist groups hope that newly registered voters will remember them with favor and support their agendas and candidates on election day.

---

*Those states were Alaska, Arizona, Colorado, Delaware, Hawaii, Idaho, Iowa, Kansas, Maine, Michigan, Minnesota, Nevada, North Dakota, South Carolina, Utah, Vermont, Washington, and Wyoming.

In 1984 the political action committee (PAC) of the Maryland Nurses' Association (MNA), then called Nurses United for Responsible State Elections (NURSE), set as its goal the registration of at least 80% of Maryland's registered nurses by 1986. The leaders knew that it is always easier to elect people who understand health care issues than to educate those people after they are elected. They believed that nurses' votes would help elect state officials sympathetic to nursing and its positions on health policy. (We will have much more to say about PACs in Chapter 8.)

A member from each MNA district became an informational resource. And the MNA newspaper, *The Maryland Nurse,* published rallying calls for voter registration, nurse participation in the political process, and the names, addresses, and phone numbers of the district PAC representatives.

The MNA's Prince George's County district association organized a voter registration day at the county's largest hospital. The original goal was to register nurses and hospital personnel, but as the day went on hospital visitors and patients were also registered. The nursing organizers concluded that all of these people have a special stake in health care.

Lois Neuman, chairwoman of the Prince George's Community College Department of Nursing at the time, served as her district's NURSE liaison. She, Ann Lombardi, a registered nurse and elected member of the Prince George's County Council, and Dianne Bukoski, a childbirth educator, organized the effort. Neuman describes the group's activities in this way:

> Ann, Dianne, and I had worked effectively together on a number of projects. Dianne and I had been district nurses' association (DNA) presidents, and Ann's knowledge and entree to county politics made us a good working team. We knew that nurses are busy people, so we wanted to accomplish our goal with minimum effort.
>
> The three of us divided the organizational tasks. The board of elections required that one of us take a one-hour course to learn the rules, regulations, and legalities of how one registers someone to vote. Ann was a natural choice for this job. She took the course. She was at the hospital all day to sign off registration forms and to answer questions raised by both nurses and registrants. Then she hand-delivered the filled-out forms to the board of elections office so that nothing was left to chance.
>
> Dianne lined up the nurses to act as registrars and scheduled their time. She divided the time we expected to work into two-hour blocks and made sure that two nurses were on duty at all times. She also planned ways to make our tables eye-catching. She brought cardboard, Magic Markers, Scotch tape, and helium balloons.
>
> I made the arrangements with the hospital: obtained permission; arranged for tables, space, and security; and wrote stories to publicize the day for both the hospital and our district nurses' association newsletter.
>
> Our registration centers opened at 6:30 AM. Our goal was to reach the maximum number of people. We were open at the change of every shift, during visiting hours, and during all of the intervening hours.
>
> One attractively decorated table was set up near the hospital's information desk near the garage—in the area of heaviest traffic. Another was set up at the change of shifts outside the office where people pick up their paychecks. We specifi-

cally made payday "registration day," believing that on that day we had the best chance to reach the most hospital employees.

While our original goal had been to register nurses, as the day went on we did a brisk business in registering other hospital personnel and visitors. Our table attracted interest. Nurses are non-threatening; people felt comfortable approaching us to ask questions not only about registering but about polling places, candidates, and the voting process. We stationed nurses in the public areas of the hospital. In a non-pressured way we invited people to register. Ann in her charismatic way was especially effective.

We had asked the hospital for permission to approach patients about registering. Permission was granted, but too late for us to organize to do it. Our intention was to ask from the door if a patient were interested and to enter the room only on invitation. Other nurses setting up registration drives might consider targeting these potential registrants.

Advance publicity about the drive had been highlighted in both the hospital and the DNA newsletter. Hospital personnel knew we were coming. After the drive we thanked—both personally and through the newsletters—everyone who had helped make the drive a success.

Our effort was completely non-partisan. We did not endorse candidates. But we did stimulate interest in voter participation. At day's end we had registered 225 potential voters. Hospital and nursing administrators, security guards, visitors, housekeeping personnel, and others thanked us.

The effort provided a public service, gave nurses visibility in the community, and projected a very positive image of nursing.[6]

PREPARE TO VOTE

Every citizen has the right and the responsibility to vote thoughtfully. History is filled with stories of how one vote, or a few, made the difference. The box below lists a few of them. Your vote counts, so use it wisely.

How Important is One Vote?

In 1645 one vote gave Oliver Cromwell control of England.

In 1649 one vote caused Charles I of England to be executed.

In 1776 one vote gave America the English language instead of German.

In 1845 one vote brought Texas into the Union.

In 1868 one vote saved President Andrew Johnson from impeachment.

In 1875 one vote changed France from a monarchy to a republic.

In 1876 one vote gave Rutherford B. Hayes the presidency of the United States.

In 1923 one vote gave Adolf Hitler leadership of the Nazi Party.

In 1941 one vote saved Selective Service—just weeks before Pearl Harbor was attacked.

Author unknown

There are many ways to inform yourself. Newspapers, magazines, and television cover the issues and the candidates. Interview programs give office seekers opportunities to present their points of view. Local cable television stations feature programs dealing with community issues. A number of organizations sponsor "meet the candidates" forums. Some are very informal: invitational and possibly held in someone's living room. Other, more structured forums are advertised, held in a public place, and open to everyone.

The League of Women Voters

The League of Women Voters, an independent, non-partisan women's organization, is dedicated to public education on political issues and candidates. In existence since 1920, the League studies issues, informs voters, and in some localities sponsors "meet the candidates" nights. It has a reputation for fairness and responsibility. Many nurses have acquired their basic education and training in political work through participation in League activities.

In recent years the League has sponsored televised debates between the candidates, starting with precedent-setting debates between presidential candidates John F. Kennedy and Richard M. Nixon in 1960. Since that time Americans, in the comfort of their living rooms, have been able to see debates between major contenders for the presidency. In 1988 the League and other groups sponsored a number of televised debates during the primaries. In these debates, presidential hopefuls from one party debated with each other: Democrats with Democrats and Republicans with Republicans. Every citizen with a television set had a special opportunity to size up the candidates, at least within the limits of this exposure.

In addition, in many communities the League publishes a comprehensive voter guide before each election. In it candidates' backgrounds are profiled and their answers to two or three key questions on the issues are recorded. Such guides may be inserted in local papers and/or are available in libraries and other public places. Many newspapers provide a similar service. The League does not endorse candidates, but other organizations, including nurse PACs, as well as newspapers frequently do. Voters are free to agree or disagree with these endorsements. But they are influential and are valued by politicians.

Boards of Elections

Boards of elections frequently send out unmarked sample ballots. In addition political parties and candidates sometimes mail them to members of their party, but theirs are marked to highlight their candidates. The samples in both cases are designed to look like the ballots used in the voting booth. Once you have studied the candidates, you can mark a sample ballot according to your conscience and take it with you for reference when you actually vote.

• • •

When you cast your ballot in the general election, you may decide to vote a straight ticket, for example, Democrat or Republican. Or you may prefer to "split your ticket," making your choices for certain offices on an individual rather than a party basis. This individual selection is often done and is the reason the nation or a state may elect an executive, president or governor, from one party and a majority in a legislative body from the other. If your ballot is especially long, confidence in your party may help you make decisions about candidates for lesser offices.

GETTING INVOLVED IN YOUR POLITICAL PARTY

For many voting may be their greatest contribution to their party. But once informed on the issues and candidates, you may decide, as I did, to become involved in party activities. A call to your party's headquarters will give you information about its organizational structure and volunteer activities.

Legislative districts are divided into *precincts* or *wards,* the smallest political division. Boundaries are set by the local board of elections supervisors. I started my public political career as a Democratic Party precinct worker in my neighborhood.

Approximately 2,000 people, Democrats and Republicans, live within the boundaries of my precinct. My experience as a precinct worker gave me a wonderful opportunity to get acquainted with the people in my neighborhood. It was a social as well as a political activity; it meant meeting new people, being sure they were registered to vote, distributing voter information in the precinct, collecting "Dollars for Democrats" (a fund-raising effort for party activities on the precinct and county levels), and holding a "meet the candidates" coffee hour in my home.

When the precinct chairman (sometimes called "captain") resigned, I was asked to run for that office—and was elected. (In some districts, precinct organizers are appointed by party leaders.) In this position my duties expanded. I appointed a vice-chairperson, treasurer, and block captains, and we planned strategy with other precinct workers. We handled fund raising for the state and local party organization in the precinct and kept people in our neighborhood informed through a newsletter.

My Republican counterpart and I were responsible for staffing the polling place with judges on election days. Each of us submitted the names of a number of candidates for the position to the county board of elections supervisors. From our lists an equal number of Democratic and Republican judges were appointed. Precinct chairs are also responsible for seeing that campaign workers at the polls abide by election laws. For example, one such law is that campaigning must stop within a designated distance from the polling place.

By becoming involved in the precinct I became acquainted with party leadership in the county and was asked to chair the countywide "Dollars for Democrats" campaign. I took on additional activities as time went on.

My experience is typical of people who have found political work interesting and rewarding. I urge you to become involved, at least at the local level. If you are asked to do a job and you are reliable and do the job well, you will be given more responsibility.

THE HATCH ACT AND HOW IT AFFECTS NURSES

The Hatch Act is a federal law that prohibits federal workers "to take any active part in political management or in political campaigns." It was enacted to prevent political patronage from corrupting the federal bureaucracy. Nurses who work in federal systems such as the Veterans' Administration or the military services are affected by this law. The law also covers people who work in state or local programs that receive federal funding, but the restrictions on their activities are not as stringent. In both cases certain political activities are allowed. If you think the Hatch Act may apply to you, you may find out about the limits of your political participation by writing the Office of Special Counsel, U.S. Merit Systems Protection Board, 1120 Vermont Ave. N.W., Washington, D.C. 20005.

GETTING INVOLVED IN A POLITICAL CAMPAIGN

Another avenue of political involvement is volunteering to work in a political campaign. You may do so through progression through the ranks in a party, or you may select a candidate whose philosophy most clearly reflects yours, and offer to help.

Every campaign needs money, but in local campaigns, volunteers may be even more important. In every campaign there are myriad tasks, and every one of them is necessary to the effort. These tasks can be tailored to volunteers' talents, available time, and commitment.

Here are a few that may appeal to you: campaigning door-to-door, either with a candidate or on your own; passing out literature in a neighborhood, shopping center, or mall; giving a "meet the candidate" coffee hour in your home; working in campaign headquarters stuffing envelopes, answering the phones, or preparing mailings; making calls from a phone bank urging people to come out to vote for your candidate; or running errands.

If you have the time and the commitment, there are position papers to be written and opportunities to take part in strategic planning. The thing to remember is that in every campaign there are jobs at every level, and every one of them is vital to success. (See Appendix B, Volunteer/campaign job match-up.)

An axiom of American politics is that "all politics is local." The local arena is the place in which you can probably make the most difference. Consider working for local candidates for the school board, county council, or state legislature. Your own community is the most convenient and in many ways the most satisfying place to work. Through this experience you will become acquainted with not only your neighbors but also the people who attempt to resolve your community's problems.

What rewards can you expect from this involvement? You will have begun to establish a network of like-minded people in your neighborhood and in the broader community. If your candidate is elected, you will know a policymaker to whom you can address problems. These may include nursing or health-policy issues, which the elected official may be able to influence. You will have a sense that, whether your candidate wins or loses, you have done what you could to influence the outcome of the election. Issues will have been raised and discussed. You will have made a difference.

NETWORKING

Just as nets consist of ropes or wires crossing and secured at regular intervals, so networks consist of individuals or groups who form an interrelated or interconnected chain. Networks have become indispensable vehicles for people concerned about the same issues to exchange information, gather support, and effect change. They may be formed for professional, political, social, personal, or other reasons. "Old boy networks" (usually made up of men who attended the same schools) are legendary. Women, without calling their associations "networks," have traditionally found other women a source of support in community efforts. What is comparatively new is that women are using the term *networks* and using them in a systematic way to make things happen politically.

All of the professional nursing organizations are examples of working networks. Through them we have opportunities to learn new skills, share information, communicate our professional concerns, and work for resolution of common professional problems.

"Telephone trees" are examples of the effectiveness of well-organized networks. They represent a systematic and practical method of getting information to a large number of people quickly without putting unreasonable burden on one or two persons. Each person in the network has the names and telephone numbers of several, let's say five, others. The person with the message calls her five contacts; they in turn call five more, who each call an additional five. Within a short time, the message has gone to 125 people. If the purpose of the original call had been to inform, the news is out. If the purpose had been a call to action, one could expect quick response.

Telephone trees are used effectively by the ANA and its state and district constituents—especially when the organization at any level wants support for a legislative position. On the national level the ANA calls legislative-liaison nurses in the states, who in turn call their district counterparts. On the state level, state nurses' association (SNA) representatives call contacts. A large number of nurses can be organized very quickly to write or telephone their legislators in support of nursing's position. If necessary they can be counted on to appear at the national or state capitols to lobby in person.

BUILDING COALITIONS

Networking and building coalitions have much in common. Coalitions link organizations that have a mutual interest in an issue. By combining their efforts they all gain political clout. Coalitions may be permanent alliances, or they may be formed temporarily to deal with a specific issue.

Nursing organizations are increasing their sophistication in building coalitions among themselves to deal with professional issues. An outstanding example of nursing organizations' working together occurred in response to the crisis generated when the major provider of malpractice insurance for nurse-midwives abruptly announced the termination of their coverage in July 1985.

The ANA and 22 specialty organizations in nursing joined the Nurses' Association of American College of Obstetricians and Gynecologists (NAACOG) and the American College of Nurse-Midwives (ACNM) in placing a half-page advertisement in *The Washington Post* on September 10, 1985. In it they appealed to legislators for emergency federal legislation to relieve the crisis.

They further strengthened their campaign with direct nurse-to-legislator appeals on Capitol Hill the day the advertisement appeared in the newspaper.

While the eventual resolution of the midwives' problem was not achieved through legislation, the united front demonstrated by the nursing coalition caught the attention of both Congress and the public. The nurse-midwives were not put out of business. Nursing organizations—working together—had contributed to the solution of a professional nursing problem.

Since nursing's primary interest is health care delivery, there are opportunities for coalition building with groups that share our concern on issues such as improved access to health care, standards for long-term care facilities, health care-cost containment, health care for the homeless, daily care for the homeless, the prevention of AIDS and care for its victims, and adult and child day care.

In addition, women's organizations, such as NOW, have found the ANA a natural ally on issues such as the Equal Rights Amendment, pay equity, and comparable worth.

We must seek out other groups with whom we can work on issues of mutual concern. Most communities publish lists of the organizations in the area. These lists may be found in local libraries or may be available through your county information office. By pooling our resources with others', we increase our effectiveness.

In our community a coalition of women's organizations sponsors a Montgomery County Women's Day every spring. Speakers sponsored by different groups address a variety of topics of special interest to women. Organizations set up tables to publicize their work. Our district nurses' association sets up one of them. We offer free blood pressure screening as a public service and as an enticement for women to stop and talk with us about health concerns.

Copies of our *Directory of Nurses in Private Practice, Health Care Services,* a DNA project, are available to any interested person. The directory serves three purposes: it informs the public about the services nurses provide in the county, advertises these services (a help to the nurse-entrepreneur), and increases public awareness about what nurses in advanced practice do.

The event also provides an opportunity to let other organizations know about our speakers bureau, through which nurses are available to speak to community groups on health and health-policy matters.

Events such as Women's Day give nursing organizations visibility among women's groups with whom coalitions may be mutually beneficial.

It is important that nurses be on the planning committees for all such events. If not asked to participate, nursing organizations should volunteer to send a representative.

YOU *WILL* MAKE A DIFFERENCE

Participation is the key to a viable democracy. We have seen how hard and long dedicated people have struggled to broaden enfranchisement in this country. Their assumption has been that given the vote, people will exercise their will for the benefit of all.

Whether or not you become involved in the political process, you will make a difference. The people who default on their responsibilities as citizens also influence. When no more than half the electorate turns out to vote, the small number of people who do vote exercise unfair power. Their candidates and positions on issues may not represent the will of the majority, but they will prevail if the majority fails to register its views.

Some people believe that media projections influence voters. Remember that elections are decided by voters, not by pollsters. Regardless of predictions by the so-called experts—whether your candidate is favored to win or projected to lose—your vote is important. Voters frequently prove the experts wrong.

Sometimes, especially when you have to vote late on election day, you may think, "The election has already been decided, so why vote?" As they say in sports, "It ain't over until it's over." Your vote cast 5 minutes before the polls close is just as valuable as one cast mid-morning.

We urge you at least to inform yourself on the issues and candidates and to vote in every election.

Nurses are naturals for political work. We have the organization and communication skills to be effective. Beyond voting, there are many ways for us to become involved in the political process. Each of the pieces in the process—no matter how big or small—is important. Most of us have to tailor our participation to our other commitments, which vary through the years. You may find being a precinct worker fits your schedule when you are at home with young children. Handing out campaign literature in your neighborhood or at shopping centers can be done on free weekends. If you have days off in the middle of the week, working at campaign headquarters may be right for you. If you have expertise on an issue, you may be able to write position papers at home. In short there is a job for everyone. Just as when you throw a pebble into a pond and the circles widen concentrically, so will your influence.

REFERENCES

1. Smeal E: Why and how women will elect the next president, New York, 1984, Harper & Row, Publishers, Inc.
2. Archer SE and Goehner PA: Nurses: a political force, Monterey, Calif, 1982, Wadsworth, Inc.
3. Berke RL: 50.16% voter turnout—lowest since 1924, New York Times, Dec. 17, 1988.
4. Skidmore MJ and Tripp MC: American government: a brief introduction, ed 4, New York, 1985, St. Martin's Press, Inc.
5. Kimberling W and Flor A: Federal election statistics, Tech Rep 1, Washington, DC, July 1988, FEC Clearinghouse on Election Administration.
6. Neuman L: Personal communication, March 1988.

ADDITIONAL READINGS

Brogan H: The longman history of the United States of America, New York, 1985, William Morrow & Co, Inc.
Morison SE, Commager HS, and Leuchtenkirg WE: the growth of the American republic, ed 7, New York, 1980, Oxford University Press, Inc.
Stanton EC: History of woman suffrage (1848-1861), Salem, NH, 1969, Arno Press, Inc.
Wollstonecraft M: A vindication of the rights of women, New York, 1967, WW Norton & Co, Inc.

Chapter 4

⚡ NURSING'S IMAGE AND HOW TO INFLUENCE IT

Nursing's image became a major professional interest in the 1980s, when it was intensively studied, written about, and discussed. But it was a study of the acute, nationwide nursing shortage in 1988 linking negative nursing images to declining nursing-school enrollments and to the problems of recruitment and retention that focused both the profession's and the public's attention on the seriousness of the problem.

In a widely publicized report issued in December 1988, a federal Commission on Nursing appointed by Otis R. Bowen, MD, Secretary of the U.S. Department of Health and Human Services, cited a negative public image of nursing as "a long-term professional liability." The commission called it "both a contributing factor to and a consequence of the current shortage."[1] The blue-ribbon, 19-member commission was chaired by Carolyne K. Davis, RN, PhD. The commission had looked into the causes of the shortage and then made recommendations for both the short- and long-term alleviation of it. While most of its proposals dealt with ways to improve the environments in which nurses work, their compensation and education, and the utilization of their skills, one of its recommendations charged the profession itself with the task of improving nursing's image.

This chapter considers the apparent gap between media representations and the realities of nursing practice, how we as individuals can educate the public about what we do, and a few examples of what some nursing organizations have done to enhance the profession's image. We'll talk briefly about changes in nursing practice that are keys to improving nursing's image and cite a few institutions that have found innovative ways to attract and retain nurses. We'll talk about the importance of convincing legislators and others in policy-making positions that nursing has a vital interest in health care delivery and about whether organized nursing's entrance into the political arena has in fact had a positive influence on the profession's image.

Since the 1850s nurses have wrestled with the dichotomy of being seen as saints on one hand, sinners on the other. No nurse before or since has been a more effective image maker than Florence Nightingale. In her lifetime she shaped nursing to fit the vision of what she thought it should be. She changed the public's perception of the women who cared for the sick away from that of Sarry Gamp, the wretched hired "nurse" in Charles Dickens' novel *Martin Chuzzlewit,* to that of trained and disciplined practitioners of the nursing arts. Nightingale realized that if people of intelligence and good character were to be attracted to the embryonic profession, nursing must be perceived as respectable. And through her example, her worldwide prestige, her determination, and her persuasive writing, she made it so.

Still, more than 80 years after Nightingale's death, the problem of nursing's image is not wholly resolved. Perhaps it is because as the profession has matured, we nurses have heightened expectations. We want nursing to be seen as respected—not just respectable.

MEDIA IMAGE

In the 1980s the husband and wife research team of Philip A. and Beatrice J. Kalisch extensively studied the image of nurses and the nursing profession as portrayed in television, movies, novels, and the press. They were widely published and became much-sought speakers by nursing groups around the country. They pointed out that these images influence not only the public's perception of nursing but also nurses' perceptions of themselves.

Given the vagueness with which most lay people perceive what nurses do, exposure to television and movie images is bound to make a difference, particularly for young people. It is estimated that the average teenager graduating from high school has spent more time watching television (15,000 hours) than in school (12,000). Twelve to twenty-year-olds make up 41% of movie-theater audiences. The opportunity to view movies at home on videotapes surely has increased their exposure to this medium. These young people are in the age group most likely to choose nursing as a career. Unfavorable entertainment-media presentations of nursing, therefore, are damaging to our efforts to attract bright, capable students to nursing.

The Kalisches believe that nursing's image as projected in the media has far-reaching consequences on health care policy decisions. They have concluded that on all political levels—local, state, and federal—there are limited health care funds to be dispersed and that the allocation of scarce resources for the delivery of nursing services is related to the media's ability to make nursing important in the public consciousness.[2]

UNRECOGNIZED SUPPORT

Curiously, in spite of the Kalisches' thorough documentation of the many negative, or what they call "non-entity," presentations of nurses by today's entertainment media, at least two studies have shown that the public has a high regard for nurses.

One was the Fingerhut-Granados study, done for the ANA in 1985. The group surveyed attitudes regarding nursing and health care issues as reflected by a national random sample of 602 adults. In addition, it tested the attitudes of 151 professionals in the print and electronic media.

The most important findings of the study were that both groups of respondents believed that nurses can play a larger role as health providers, that nurses "probably have good ideas on how to reduce the costs of health care," and that enlarging their responsibilities could help contain health care costs.

"In noneconomic areas," the report stated, "nurses were found to be better at ensuring quality in the 'intangibles' of health care such as personal and emotional needs of patients." These included clarification for patients and their families of exactly what a doctor says and seeing to it that patients eat properly and are treated humanely.

The survey also revealed that "the greater the amount of time the media professional spent covering health-related issues, the more supportive that respondent was to an expansion of the health care role of nurses."[3]

In 1988 Nancy Wiederhorn, RN, DNSc, a professor of nursing at George Mason University in Fairfax, Va., made public data that she had collected regarding the public's attitudes about nursing and nurses' perceptions of themselves. Using standardized tests to measure attitudes, she surveyed two groups at a northeastern university during the 1986-1987 and 1987-1988 school years. One group, which Wiederhorn considered representative of the public, was made up of those attending university open houses. It consisted of 177 prospective university students (those considering all disciplines) and their families. The second group was made up of 216 students in advanced undergraduate nursing classes. When asked to rank different occupations in terms of "most desirable," both groups ranked "nurse" higher than all others, including social worker, teacher, physician, engineer, lawyer, or average woman. Most occupations were ranked significantly lower than nursing.

In contrast to a common perception that nurses suffer from poor self-esteem, the nurses in this study ranked themselves significantly higher than other professionals. "My data shows that, among the people I surveyed, nurses are regarded as exemplary people—high in wisdom, intellect, sincerity, strength, dependability, and warmth," says Wiederhorn. "This suggests that nursing must look at factors other than image as the cause of declining nursing school enrollments."[4]

EVERY NURSE'S PERSONAL RESPONSIBILITY FOR THE IMAGE

While these two studies document the perception that nurses have accrued an immense amount of goodwill with the public, most nurses believe that our image as health professionals needs improvement. We registered nurses in the United States number approximately 2 million strong. Everyone knows a nurse—as a relative, a friend, or a neighbor. What is troubling, however, is that few people understand the role of today's nurse in our health care delivery system. Few people have a clear idea of what nurses do, the preparation required for different kinds of practice, or nursing's steady advance toward professionalism in recent years.

While media images are important, people's most vivid perceptions come from personal experience. People meet us in our work place, in community activities, and in social situations. We nurses are most responsible for nursing's image. It is up to us to make our professional and personal contacts with the public positive ones.

Patients and their families are acutely aware of nurses. Those who provide direct patient care—no matter what their practice setting—make the most vivid impressions on the public. What they see us doing in practice, however, is a very incomplete picture of nursing.

Patients do not actually see nurses assessing their physical and emotional status, drawing conclusions on the basis of sophisticated education, and taking appropriate actions to prevent complications or to remedy present problems. They may feel the psychological support the nurse provides and may appreciate the health teaching she or he gives, but they are probably not thinking about these services. Most often they do not realize that these intangibles are part of professional nursing. In some cases we will have to attempt to explain them.

Addressing the difficulty of explaining nurses' intangible services, Mary B. Mallison, RN, editor of the American Journal of Nursing, focused in a September 1987 editorial on how nurses can better represent themselves to the media. She said, "It's not easy to describe what we do, but it's not impossible, either." Mallison had specific suggestions on how to do it that are as useful in explaining nursing to a patient or a legislator as to a media representative. She said:

> Suppose you work on a surgical floor and your local TV or newspaper reporter challenges you with, "I've been a patient here. After surgery, don't nurses mostly just change dressings and give antibiotics and painkillers and—pass bedpans?"
>
> "Oh, yes," you answer. "We change dressings. In doing so, we keep watch over how wounds heal or deteriorate, and we change (or persuade the surgeon to change) strategies accordingly. We decide how to position you for comfort and safety and in ways that prevent complications of breathing, circulation, and digestion. We help you look at your own wound and begin to accept it as part of yourself, but not the most important part. We affirm your wholeness as a person by the way we look at you, touch you, and respond to you. We teach you to see signs of healing, so that you keep getting booster shots of encouragement.
>
> "Oh, yes, we do give painkillers and antibiotics. Lots of them, mostly into your veins. We have to know how fast or slowly to give them, and when is the best time, and how soon they are likely to leave your bloodstream, and whether or not they'll interact strangely with your other medicines, and what their bad effects will look like in you.
>
> "And have you wondered why we're always draped with stethoscopes? There's a good reason. We're often listening to your lungs and bowels, both slowed down by anesthesia and surgery. And we're listening to your heartbeat and blood pressure for signs of internal bleeding. . . .

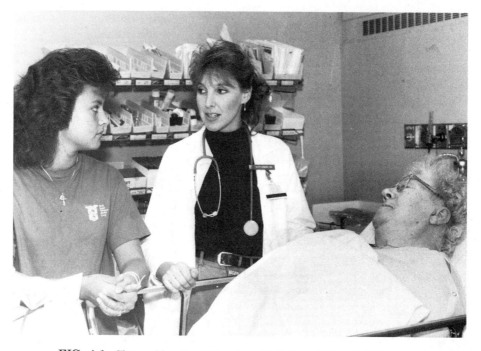

FIG. 4-1. Choose Nursing! (Courtesy Beth Israel Hospital, Boston.)

"Then we verify our observations by checking your lab values. And on the way to the desk, where we'll arrange for the services and supplies you'll continue to need at home . . . we also empty your bedpan."[5]

WHAT ORGANIZATIONS CAN DO TO ENHANCE NURSING'S IMAGE

The profession's growing interest in its image has spurred different kinds of nursing organizations to action. While there must be others equally valuable, let's look at a few comparatively small-scale efforts that could be duplicated in any community.

Janet A. Secatore, program specialist at the Center for the Advancement of Nursing Practice at Beth Israel Hospital in Boston, Mass., describes their community outreach and career awareness program called "Choose Nursing!" Working with high school science teachers, nurses from Beth Israel, in collaboration with the volunteer services and community relations department, have established school-hospital partnerships. Each month high school faculty and students visit the hospital for a day and are paired with nurses as they care for patients (Fig. 4-1). Partnerships are extended to six weeks during the summer.

One-day visitors are given bright-blue T-shirts marked "Volunteer," and summer partners wear lab coats, so that students are clearly identifiable.

Volunteer nurses are selected on the basis of their professionalism and their enthusiasm for the program. In the 2 years the program has been in existence, 150 students have had a first-hand opportunity to learn what nursing actually is. The program has received coverage on both ABC and NBC news, as well as a grant from the Mabel A. Horne Trust, administered by The Bank of Boston.

Secatore says nurses and students like the program. "Nurses," she says, "feel that they are making a personal contribution to the improvement of nursing's image."

She cautions, however, that nurses may not receive a positive response among teachers in every high school. "If the first school you try is not interested, try others until you get a fit," she says.[6]

Another community effort involved the public relations committee of our DNA, which reserved display space in three public libraries for the month of May 1989. Using the ANA's theme for that year's Nurses' Day, "Nurses Change Lives," cases and bulletin boards were filled with recruitment posters, attractive pictures of nurses caring for patients, and a flier encouraging the viewer to seek more information about a nursing career. The names and telephone numbers of our DNA president and of the chairpersons of the two nursing programs in the county were included. Other nursing organizations were invited to provide exhibit materials and were credited as contributors to the displays.

A Girl Scout troop, in which one of the DNA board members had a daughter, assisted in the development of a display in a particularly awkward space. It was a horizontal glass cabinet that was approximately 4 feet square. Working with nurses the girls made a diorama showing the settings in which nurses work. Buildings representing hospitals, nursing homes, a research center, schools, a birthing center, homes, industry, and a prison were made from different-sized medicine boxes covered with contact paper and decorated appropriately.

Local newspapers and television stations were notified well in advance of the exhibits' openings. They were advised that the displays represented photo opportunities and that stories could be pegged on National Nurses' Day. (We will talk more about working with the media in the next chapter.)

A public forum was held at one of the libraries on a Saturday afternoon. Again using the theme "Nurses Change Lives," nurses from different practice disciplines, such as hospital nursing, education, midwifery, and enterostomal therapy, gave brief talks illustrating the breadth of nursing practice. Time was set aside for questions, a nursing recruitment video, and refreshments.

Organizers of the image-enhancing promotion were pleased with it for several reasons. The attention-getting exhibits were situated in highly visible locations. Public libraries are busy places frequented by people of all ages. In each library the display was up for one month. Once the materials were assembled, exhibits could be moved to another of the county's 23 libraries, thereby multiplying their effectiveness by making them visible to different audiences. The effort was a cooperative one involving nurses in a number of nursing organizations in the county. Finally, by involving members of a youth group, nurses exposed them in an informal way to valid information about nursing as a career.

The nursing organizations of Baltimore city and county collaborate each year in sponsoring a Nurses' Day celebration in a public place where pedestrian traffic is heavy. For many years the event was held at the Baltimore Civic Center. Local public officials were invited to be on the speakers' stand when outstanding nurse awards were given. Contributing groups made attractively displayed information on nursing and health available to the public, and nurses were there to answer questions regarding wide-ranging subjects such as high blood pressure, cancer, and educational opportunities in nursing.

Several nursing organizations have established speakers bureaus. Set up at either state or local levels, they facilitate dissemination of nursing's message to the public. Attractive, articulate nurses, whether they are speaking on health or nursing issues, can do much to impress community groups with our professionalism. Organizers should try to arrange for nurses to speak to high school counselors and science teachers about nursing careers. Local television and radio stations should be advised of the availability of nurses to appear as experts when news demands the comments of a health professional.

IMPROVE NURSING PRACTICE—IMPROVE NURSING'S IMAGE

Perhaps we all come into nursing with some idealized expectations about it. Most of us maintain this vision through school—and beyond—or we would not stay. However, when we consider reality as it relates to nursing's image, we must ask, "Does nursing as it is practiced meet our own ideals? If it does not, how can we improve the practice?"

Many nurses believe that a key to changing the image of nursing is change in the practice of nursing. One such nurse is Myrtle K. Aydelotte, RN, PhD, a professor emeritus at the College of Nursing, University of Iowa. She has said, "In most settings . . . nurses are not granted the privilege of control of their own practice. Within most institutions, the staff nurse plays a limited part in determining policies relating to practice and self-governance."[7]

More than 68% of employed nurses work in hospitals.[8] We can assume that the majority of hospital nurses are employed at the staff level. When underrecognized and overworked, these nurses (particularly those working on non–high-tech units) often suffer from low morale and poor self-esteem, two negative factors when it comes to projecting a positive image. Ultimately, any system that improves working conditions, expands opportunities for educational advancement, increases salaries, and involves rank-and-file nurses in making the policies that affect their practice will improve nursing's image.

In some practice settings collective bargaining has provided an avenue for some staff nurses to influence decisions that affect their work environments.

Contracts hammered out between hospital managers and nursing unions reflect rank-and-file nurses' interest in issues involving their practice. Such issues include safe nurse/patient ratios, release from non-nursing functions, and opportunities for staff nurses to take part in formulating policy that affects their work. In some situations these issues are perceived as more important than salary increases and benefit plans.

Even in 1988, at the peak of the nursing shortage, some hospital nurse-managers, cognizant of the need for recognition of staff nurses, were able to organize the way nursing was practiced in their institutions so that excellence was rewarded and nurses attracted and retained.

One such nurse-manager was Joyce Clifford, vice-president for nursing at Beth Israel Hospital in Boston. In January 1988, during the height of the nursing shortage, vacancies of 13% to 14% were common in many hospitals. At Beth Israel they were 2%. There the whole organization was set up to support and protect the primary nursing relationship. Clifford said, "We try to give the people at the bedside the skills, the ability, and the support to solve a problem, whether a conflict or a clinical question, where it occurs. We don't ask them to call people in to do it for them; we ask them to call people in to help them solve it." Susan Kilroy, a clinical adviser, said, "Staff nurses know their patients. . . . Everyone—the whole health care team—respects the primary nurse for what she knows."

Other staff-nurse–centered approaches to hospital-nursing management have been highly successful in places such as Newark Beth Israel Medical Center in New Jersey, the Henry May Newhall Memorial Hospital in Valencia, Calif., the Santa Monica Hospital in Santa Monica, Calif.,[9] and the Rush/Presbyterian/ St. Luke's Medical Center in Chicago,[10] to name a few.

The Secretary's Commission on Nursing studied 11 other hospitals around the country that had developed and implemented successful strategies for the recruitment and retention of nurses. It found that they all shared common elements, which included management commitment to nursing and nurses, strong nursing leadership, and competitive salaries and benefits. Nursing leadership focused on strategic planning, commitment to patient care, decentralized decision-making, nurses' involvement in decision-making, problem identification and solution, commitment to education, and employee recognition.[11]

Janice M. Feldman, vice-president for nursing at the New Rochelle Medical Center, New Rochelle, N.Y., and former director of nursing at the Warren Magnuson Clinical Center of the National Institutes of Health (NIH) in Bethesda, Md., believes that both retention and recruitment are based on measures that appeal to nurses' professional pride. She also believes that recruitment advertising can educate the public and enhance nursing's image.

When she became director of nursing at the NIH Clinical Center in 1985, the staff vacancy rate was 20%. She believed that restructuring the organization, strengthening internal communication, solving problems jointly, and involving staff nurses in decision-making were vital in improving the situation.

While implementing these changes, Feldman also initiated a very successful recruitment campaign. In a series of advertisements placed in leading newspapers and magazines, the NIH emphasized the challenge of nursing, nurses' responsibilities for life and death, the opportunity to improve the quality of people's lives, and the satisfaction of caring for people.

Since NIH is a research center, Feldman focused on opportunities for nurses to be on the leading edge of new developments in medicine and nursing. She emphasized that collaborative relationships between physicians and nurses are the norm at NIH. An appeal for nurses to work in units in which AIDS is being studied read, "There's a small team in town getting ready to fight today's biggest health threat. Join us." Another appealed to oncology nurses by saying, "At NIH the world will watch what you do as a cancer nurse." "Through these ads we attempt to remind nurses of the profession's larger mission," says Feldman.

Feldman looks on these advertisements as a way to educate the public about nursing, as well as an effort to attract nurses. One of them said, "At NIH 1:4 is an everyday nurse/patient ratio." Feldman says, "We have to let the public know that ratios are important."

An ad published in national non-nursing magazines (*Time, Sports Illustrated, Science,* and *Modern Health Care*) featured an attractive nurse under a caption that read, "Kim Cox is a project manager. Kim Cox is a nurse." It also described Cox's work (Fig. 4-2).

Periodically, the hospital uses large advertisements to commend and thank its nurses. It lists by name and the units on which they work those who are owed special recognition for excellence.

As staff positions filled in late 1988, the NIH advertised, "Once again, NIH proves the exception not the rule." At a time when there were openings in almost every hospital in the country, the NIH announced that it had no more vacancies. It does maintain a waiting list.

At NIH Feldman proved that nurses can be recruited by appealing to their sense of professionalism and the positive aspects of nursing. They can be retained by ensuring good communication between management and staff and by providing opportunities for staff nurses to participate in decision-making in areas that affect their practice.

While the media's images of nursing make a difference, the practice and structure of nursing must improve if nursing's image is to get better. We must pay more attention to the needs of hospital staff nurses, who make up the majority of practicing nurses. Nursing leaders are speaking out forcefully for recognition of the vital contributions of those nurses who provide direct patient care.

Carol Lindeman, RN, PhD, FAAN, dean of the Oregon Health Sciences University in Portland, said it well in a March 1987 editorial in *The American Nurse:* "When push comes to shove, I would say our view of the staff nurse will determine the future of nursing . . . it is about time we give credit where credit is due and recognize staff nurses as the heart, head, and soul of nursing."[12]

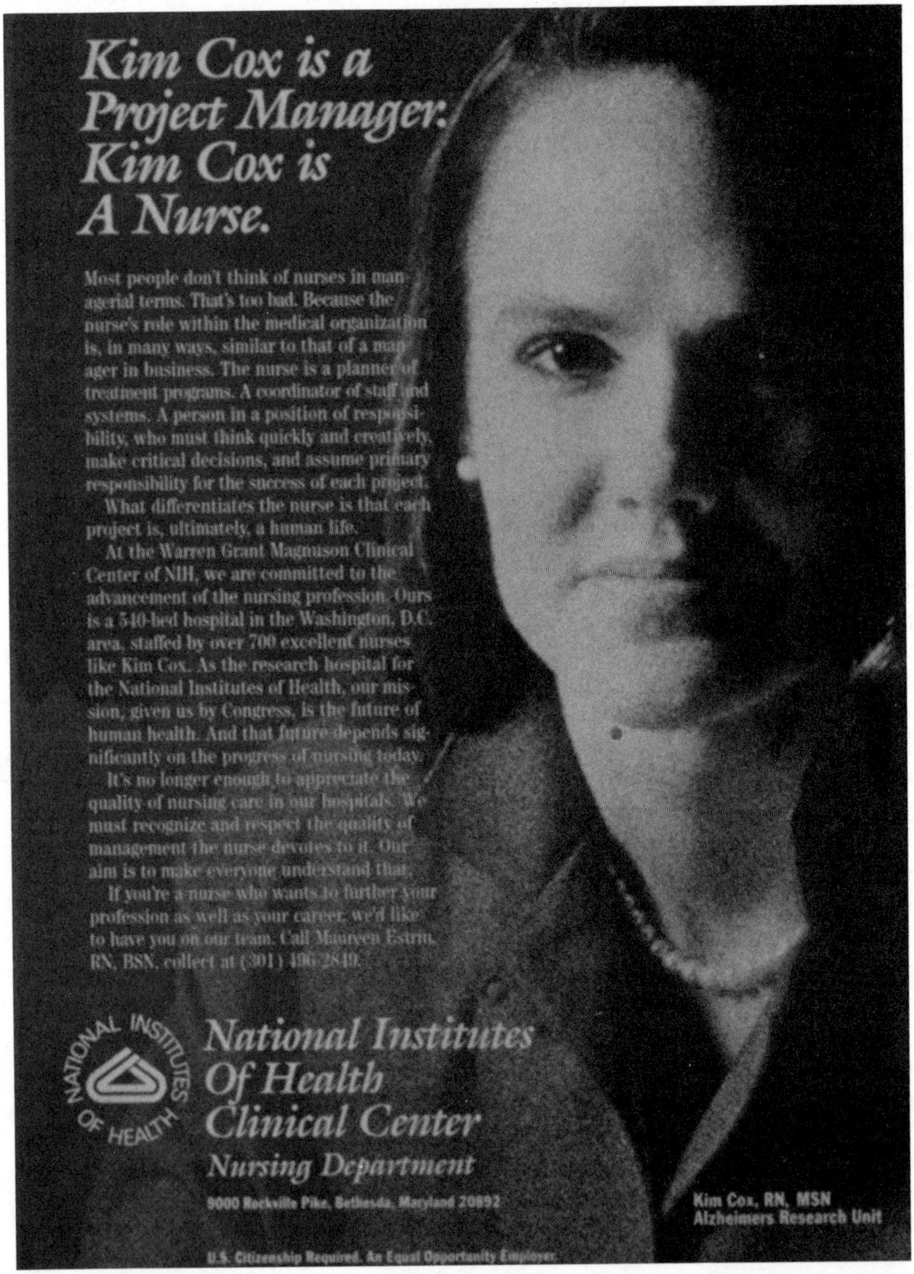

FIG. 4-2. Example of an advertisement designed to educate the public and enhance nursing's image. (Reprinted with permission of the National Institutes of Health.)

LEGISLATORS' PERSPECTIVES

Do legislators perceive nurses in any way different from the way the public sees them? And do their perceptions influence our effectiveness in attaining the health-policy goals we believe are appropriate?

As a nurse who has worked on both sides of the political fence, first as a community activist and then as a member of the Maryland General Assembly, I have learned that perceptions often have a greater effect on legislative actions than reality does. Every day, legislators deal with perceptions—of each other, the people who come to press their causes, the issues, and the impact those issues are likely to have on constituents.

In Washington, D.C., and in the state capitols, legislators perceive that the ANA and its constituent SNAs speak for the broad group of nursing interests. They assume that nursing's specialty organizations address the narrower interests of their particular practice. It is important that all nursing organizations communicate with and support each other. We must learn how to present a united front, avoiding the appearance of conflict. Advances made by one group of nurses may open the door for others.

Until recently most legislators had not thought of nurses as influential players in the political arena. Nurses, like many women, have been seen as nurturers and helpers, not power brokers. In fact, for many years because of our potential strength due to our numbers and our lack of political activity, nursing was sometimes referred to as "the sleeping giant."

Within the past 10 years, however, the ANA and its SNAs have organized, advanced a legislative agenda, and developed the sophistication that has resulted in politicians' eagerly working with the nursing profession to develop health policy. Through their PACs and those of other nursing specialists' organizations, nurses have helped elect candidates known to be friendly to our interests. Nevertheless, we are still new in the business of politics, and there is much more to be done to strengthen our political leverage.

Educating Legislators

Legislators have a great deal of respect for nurses. But they know little about the nurse's role in today's health care delivery system. It is nurses' responsibility to educate them, if we expect them to know and understand our needs and the needs of those who seek our services. We can do that even by the manner in which we introduce ourselves.

When you meet legislators, public officials, or media personnel, start by clearly identifying yourself as a registered nurse. Tell them the name of the school from which you graduated and the name of the professional organization to which you belong. Explain what you do. Show through your introduction why you have something of value to say about the measure you support. Use language that is understandable to the person with whom you are speaking. Avoid using nursing jargon, which most lay people would not readily understand. Be specific. For instance, say:

> I am Mary Jones. I am a registered nurse, a member of the Maryland Nurses' Association, and a graduate of Montgomery Community College.
> I work on an orthopedic unit, where we see many patients with broken bones. Often they are victims of accidents involving drunk drivers. I am interested in legislation that will get these drivers off the roads.

Or you might say:

> I am Susan Smith. I am a registered nurse and a graduate of the Union Memorial Hospital and the University of Maryland's Schools of Nursing. I work in the newborn intensive care unit at General Hospital. As we care for these high-risk babies, we observe them very carefully and try to identify problems that require attention. Many of these babies are what we used to call "premature." Our work is demanding, and the cost of bringing these babies to a point at which they can go home is expensive. Because we know that premature delivery is one of the causes of low birth weight in babies, I am interested in legislation that will expand prenatal-care programs for indigent women. We believe they will help reduce the number of high-risk babies.

When you have scheduled a meeting to talk with your legislator, prepare yourself to speak intelligently about the issues in which you are interested. Once a legislator realizes that you are knowledgeable, that legislator will call on you for more information about a variety of health issues. Have a business card available, one with your name, position, address, and phone number. Be sure to leave it when you offer to provide more help.

Getting to know your elected representatives in advance sets the stage for a more productive exchange when you really want support for a specific health or nursing issue. And nothing beats working in a candidate's campaign as a means of demonstrating interest. It also provides informal opportunities to get better acquainted.

Building Bridges Between Nurses and Legislators

Many SNAs have found ways to develop a closer rapport with their local legislators. In Maryland it began in this way.

As a new member of the state legislature, I was impressed with the effectiveness of the Maryland Medical Society in getting support for their positions in the General Assembly. Each year they wine and dine the legislators and give each one a list of the society's priorities for the upcoming session. Once the session is in progress, the group again invites the legislators to dinner. This time they criticize or praise them according to how they have voted on the physicians' issues.

While I seldom recommend that nurses model themselves after physicians, I suggested we borrow from them in this instance and find a social way to establish contacts that would be both effective and within our financial means.

In 1976 members of the executive board of our DNA for the first time rather timidly extended an invitation to county legislators to meet with them before the session to discuss issues of mutual concern at an informal, dutch-treat dinner.

The event was so successful that the next year I offered my home for a nurse-legislator supper. My one rule was that food must be prepared and on the table before the guests arrived. No nurses were allowed in the kitchen during the affair. I wanted them to be out talking with legislators.

Since then the event has grown into an annual reception for nurses, legislators, and elected county officials. And the practice has been duplicated in all the districts in Maryland with great success. In addition, the SNA, in collaboration with several nursing specialty groups, now sponsors a legislative reception in Annapolis, our state capital, during the legislative session. An open invitation is extended to legislators and all nurses.

In the past decade nurses in many parts of the country have become aware of the need to create opportunities for nurses and legislators to become better acquainted. SNA publications have reflected the fact that similar receptions are now relatively commonplace throughout the country.

Timing is important in planning such events. Nurse-sponsored "meet the candidates" nights before an election will bring out a crowd of office-seekers and give nurses an opportunity to size up the candidates. But if your goal is to get acquainted with the people who will be influential once the legislature is in session, it is better to wait until after the election. Your guests then will be elected officials who can actually deal with your issues. In a nonelection year, dates set for a weekend a month or two before the legislative session begins (or very early in the session any year) will probably prove most effective for district associations. We have found that having these receptions in members' homes has worked best for us. With a group of fewer than a hundred, it just seems more hospitable.

If you are planning a legislative reception at the state capital for your state association, be aware that you have competition. In recent years the number of receptions at state capitols everywhere has burgeoned. Each legislator may receive as many as four or five invitations for each weeknight during the early weeks of the session. Nurses must compete for legislators' attention with social workers, real estate organizations, and public works contractors. Nursing's planners need to get their receptions on the legislature's calendar of such events early. Later in the session the crush of legislative work may keep lawmakers on the job. Receptions planned for these weeks are less likely to be well attended. (See box on p. 52.)

Some lobbying groups spend impressive amounts of money in their efforts to influence lawmakers, while others offer simple hospitality, such as wine and cheese receptions. The elaborateness of the affair is not the important thing. But given the reality of legislators' crowded schedules, personal notes from individual nurses to their own representatives inviting them to attend nurses' receptions greatly strengthen general invitations. Elected officials respond to their constituents. A signed note saying, for example, "I live in your district and look forward to seeing you at the Maryland Nurses' Association's reception at the

Capital Parties

Here is a sample of the dinners and receptions that Maryland legislators were invited to during the first week and a half of their session.

JAN. 11
- Open house, 2 p.m.—Montgomery County Board of Realtors.
- Reception, 3 p.m.—Associated Builders and Contractors of Maryland.
- Reception, 4:30 p.m.—Cable Television Association of Maryland.
- Cocktails/dinner, 6 p.m.—Maryland Bus Association.

JAN. 12
- Reception, 6 p.m.—Women's Bar Association.
- Reception, 6 p.m.—Maryland Chamber of Commerce.
- Cocktails/dinner, 6:30 p.m.—University of Maryland Eastern Shore, Coppin State University, Bowie State University.

JAN. 16
- Reception, 5 p.m.—Maryland Chapter, National Association of Social Workers.
- Dinner, 5:30 p.m.—Maryland Restaurant Association.
- Dinner, 6 p.m.—University of Maryland School of Law.
- Reception, 6 p.m.—Lida Lee Tall Learning Resources Center.

JAN. 17
- Reception, 5:30 p.m.—Maryland Federation of the Blind.
- Cocktails/dinner, 5:30 p.m.—Maryland State Bar Association.
- Reception, 6 p.m.—Public Works Contractors Association.
- Cocktails/dinner, 6:30 p.m.—Eastern Shore Municipal League.

JAN. 19
- Reception, 6 p.m.—Maryland Bankers Association.
- Cocktails/dinner, 6 p.m.—University of Maryland College Park.

From "Social events just a function of being a MD legislator: invitations pour in as lobbyists' ranks grow. © *The Washington Post*, January 1988.

Navy Officer's Club in Annapolis between 6 and 8 PM on January 16th," is a real draw for a legislator.

To make the most of these affairs, position papers outlining association goals for the session should be given to every elected official. Written information reinforces points already made during discussions.

For these affairs to be successful, good attendance by well-prepared nurses is essential. This means that planners must do more than give a nice party. Nothing is more counterproductive to our goals than a reception for which legislators turn out and nurses do not.

Elected officials are busy people. Their interest in attending such events is

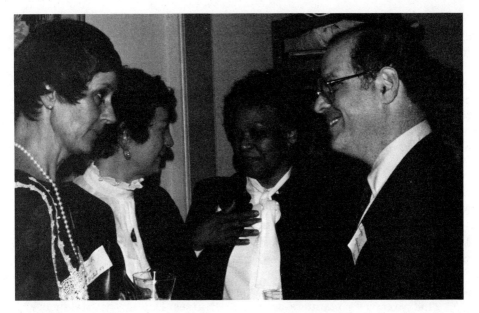

Nurses Barbara Hanley, Ada Jacox, and Lorretta Richardson discuss the issues with Maryland House Speaker Ben Cardin (now a U.S. congressman) at a "Nurses' Night" in Annapolis in January 1986.

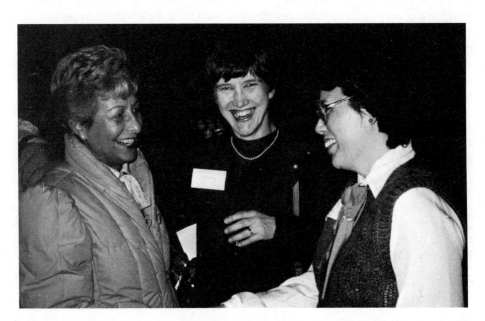

Delegate Marilyn Goldwater talks with presidents of two nursing organizations, MNA President Lynada Johnson and Maryland Emergency Room Nurses' Association President Brigid Krizek, at a "Nurses' Night" in Annapolis in January 1986.

to build support among important constituencies, so one of the images these events should project is that of nurses as a political force. Numbers play an important part in that perception.

These events should be well publicized, and nurses must be there. Telephone calls, or any other method that works, should be employed to ensure a crowd. Ideally, nurses would already be knowledgeable about the most important issues under discussion because of association meetings and articles in district and state newsletters. But even if members are not fully informed, their attendance is essential. The experience provides an opportunity to take the first step toward becoming involved in the group's political-action efforts.

NURSES' DAY AT THE STATE CAPITOL

Many other SNAs, often in collaboration with other nursing organizations, sponsor similar events. Some go a step further by sponsoring an annual "Nurses' Day" at the state capitol. One especially effective event of this kind was sponsored by the Ohio Nurses' Association (ONA) in 1985.

That year ONA planners organized "Nurses' Day at the Statehouse" to coincide with the day legislation calling for a major revision of the Ohio Nurse Practice Act was introduced. The day opened with an address by Governor Richard F. Celeste, who told the 285 assembled registered nurses, licensed practical nurses, and nursing students that his administration was proud to be part of nursing's team. The *Ohio Nurses Review,* the ONA's publication, reported that the governor "made it clear that he understands the vital role nurses have in the delivery of health care."[13]

Following the governor's remarks, ONA Legislation Committee members took 100 of the participants on a tour of the statehouse, introducing them to members of the Ohio General Assembly. Others attended educational lectures on subjects dealing with political action. Influential legislators, sitting at the head table at an ONA-sponsored luncheon, voiced their support for nursing. Representative Judy Sheerer, chief sponsor of the nurse practice act legislation, described major revisions and urged nurses to work for support of the bill in their districts.

A wine and cheese reception for legislators and nurses sponsored by the ONA concluded the day's activities. By planning the day around the introduction of a particular piece of nursing legislation, the ONA strengthened support for the bill among both legislators and nurses. Nurses had been recognized, they had been informed, and they had influenced.

INFLUENCING HEALTH POLICY: A PLUS FOR NURSING'S IMAGE

It can be argued that nursing's increased assertiveness in the area of health-policy formation is in itself a plus for the profession's image. The belief that one has had an influence on events builds personal and professional confidence, which is good for nurses and nursing. Any time well-informed nurses present their case in public, they influence their audience's perception of nursing in a positive way. This is good for nursing's image.

It has been demonstrated over and over in the U.S. Congress and in state legislatures that decision-makers will listen to us if we present them with accurate information. We have first-hand knowledge of how the health care system works. We know its strengths and its weaknesses. As nurses we are our patients' best advocates. We must share this unique knowledge with our elected representatives by making ourselves more available to them as resource people.

Knowledge is power. In the health-policy arena we must conscientiously study the issues. Each piece of proposed legislation must be addressed with a responsible eye on the effect it will have on the whole health care delivery system. With knowledge and experience each of us can become a more effective communicator and advocate, and nursing will fulfill the image we hold of it.

REFERENCES

1. U.S. Department of Health and Human Services, National Center for Health Services Research and Health Care Technology Assessment: Final report: Secretary's Commission on Nursing, Hospital Studies Program, vol 1, December 1988.
2. Kalisch PA and Kalisch BJ: The changing image of the nurse, Menlo Park, Calif, 1987, Addison-Wesley Publishing Co, Inc.
3. Fingerhut V and Granados L: ANA nursing issues national attitudinal and opinion leaders survey, Washington, D.C., 1985, Fingerhut-Granados Opinion Research Co.
4. Wiederhorn N: Personal communication, May 1, 1988.
5. Mallison MB: Are you ready for Oprah Winfrey? American Journal of Nursing 87(9): 1,127, 1987.
6. Secatore J: Personal communication, March 1989.
7. Aydelotte MK: Book review: the changing image of the nurse. Image: Journal of Nursing Scholarship 19(4):214, 1987.
8. USDHHS, Health Resources and Services Administration, Bureau of Health Professions, Division of Nursing: the registered nurse population: findings from the national sample survey of registered nurses, November 1984, June 1986.
9. Scherer P: Hospitals that attract (and keep) nurses, American Journal of Nursing 88(1):34, 1988.
10. Ballman CS: Chicago job focus: the Chicago story, American Journal of Nursing 87(10):1337, 1987.
11. Secretary's Commission on Nursing: final report, vol 2, December 1988.
12. Lindeman C: Staff nurse is the heart, head, and soul of nursing, The American Nurse 19(3):4, March 1987.
13. Ohio Nurses Review: Nurses' Day: image builder for nursing, 60(4):1, April 1985.

Chapter 5

⤜ THE MEDIA—
INFLUENCING THEM,
USING THEM

If we nurses are to increase our influence on health policy, we must learn to utilize both the print and electronic media to make the public aware of nursing's interests and positions. We must encourage reporters to write positive stories about the profession. We must correct inaccurate representations. And we must learn how better to use association newsletters and other publicity to promote the profession and our legislative agendas. When working to attract positive publicity for nursing, desire is not enough. There are practical lessons that can and must be learned. Let's start with the basics.

WHAT MAKES A STORY?

Before you begin to write or promote a story, you must define it. You may ask yourself: "What story do I have to tell? Why should a reporter or an editor listen to me? How can I catch their attention? How can I dramatize this story so that it will compete with accounts of robberies, fires, and accidents on the highway?"
- Newspaper articles and television coverage, whether feature or straight news, are usually tied to a news angle.
- Nursing shortages, difficult as they are for nurses practicing in the field, provide opportunities to educate the public about who nurses are and what they do.
- Shortages are news because of the potential disruption of vital health services. Both print and electronic media throughout the country run such stories.
- The revolutionary change caused by "prospective payment" of hospital bills by both government and private insurers is news—and so is the dramatic increase in health care costs.
- Shortened hospital stays, with the accompanying implications for both patients and nurses, and the rapid growth of the home care industry are important stories.

56

• Nurses' PAC endorsements, legislative efforts, and outstanding-nurse awards provide opportunities for positive publicity.

Once you have a story idea, you will need to find the most effective way to publicize it. Since most of us have limited time and resources, how to place important information where it will be used is a pressing consideration. In most cases local newspapers and radio and television stations present the best possibilities. They are often much more receptive to news generated by DNAs than are large metropolitan news organizations.

If you are trying to place the story in a newspaper, look at several. Take a careful look at them and focus on the most important ones, the ones most likely to reach the audience you wish to attract. Where are stories such as yours placed? If it is news, the general assignment editor may be the appropriate person to approach. If the paper is large enough to have a health section, the health editor may be interested in your idea. If you are familiar enough with the paper to know which reporters do stories on certain subjects, you could call one of them. If the story is important to the profession, you may have to "sell" it to both the editor and a reporter. You will find the names of editors listed on the mastheads of many newspapers.

The news producer determines what news will be used on television. This position is similar to that of a newspaper editor. Assignment editors dispatch reporters and camera crews to cover stories. In radio the news director manages local radio newscasts.

When making the initial contact to promote your story, telephone the appropriate person. Be prepared to present your idea concisely, and say that you will follow up by sending a one-page typewritten list of facts. Keep in mind that this person is probably not familiar with your subject, so it is up to you to present it in an understandable way. Offer to provide more information upon request.

In most cases the news organization will assign its own reporter to develop the story from original sources. But it is up to you to direct the reporter to those sources. Have names (correctly spelled) and telephone numbers available when you make your call.

Kalisch and Kalisch[1] have observed that stories about nurses in clinical practice are most helpful in building positive nursing images. Articles or television news features describing nurses caring for and teaching patients in both hospitals and homes, handling sophisticated problems in intensive care units, and showing nurses in advanced practice all project nursing at its best.

For example, Jane Hansen, RN, was a staff nurse at Abbott Northwestern Hospital in Minneapolis when this photo was taken of her with her young patient, Kim Hyun-jung (Fig. 5-1). Kim had gone through an eight-month ordeal of medical complications following open heart surgery. When Kim came from Korea she spoke no English and had no family with her. Hansen's nursing care and friendship helped Kim expand beyond her limited boundaries and to recover. This photo accompanied a story published in the *Minneapolis Star and Tribune* and was reprinted by the Minnesota Nurses Association as a cover photo in the

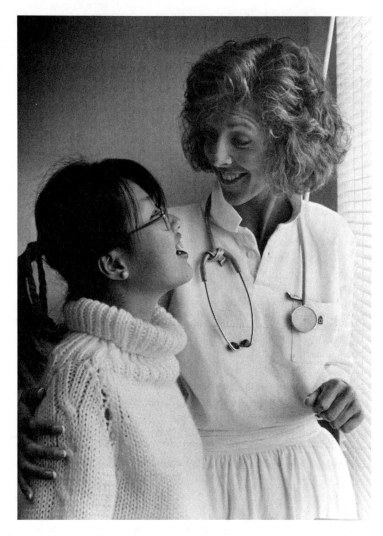

FIG. 5-1. Jane Hansen, RN, with Kim Hyun-jung. Photo courtesy of the *Minneapolis Star and Tribune,* staff photographer Rita Reed.

May 1987 *Minnesota Nursing Accent.* It is an excellent example of a photograph that projects a positive nursing image.

Some nursing associations have arranged for reporters and photographers to spend a day with a nurse. (Other associations have used the same approach to educate legislators about problems relevant to legislation under consideration.) When planning such a day, keep in mind the constraints under which your guest operates. If you can find a slow day, for example, the day after a weekly paper goes to press, you will have more of a chance for successfully promoting nursing issues.

As nurses become a scarce resource, positive stories about nurses in practice are appearing nationwide in both the print and electronic media. We can appeal to editors and producers, saying that stories that shed a positive light on nursing are in the public's interest. Nursing shortages are dangerous for the nation's health.

Once stories appear in print or on the air, we can encourage more reporting of nursing issues by sending letters thanking editors, reporters, and producers for their positive contributions.

MAKING THE MOST OF NATIONAL NURSES' DAY

The annual observation of National Nurses' Day on May 6 provides an opportunity for nursing organizations to call the public's attention to nursing and its contributions to the public good. It is an excellent time to alert the local media to opportunities for stories about nurses.

Every year the ANA develops a theme for the day and promotes its use throughout the country in order to bring national attention to the event. For example, in 1988 the ANA chose "Proud to Care" as its theme for the day. In 1989 it was "Nurses Change Lives" (Fig. 5-2).

Nevertheless, some nursing organizations prefer to develop their own ideas. For example, in 1986 the New York Mets won the World Series, and a few months later the New York Giants won the Super Bowl. New Yorkers were jubilant, to the New York State Nurses' Association chose to make a connection between nurses and the world champions. Its New York State Nurses Week poster in 1987 clearly implied that nurses are also winners (Fig. 5-3). (Note the strength of the photograph that was used: It reflects upbeat nurses—women and men—of different ages, races, and disciplines. It creates a very positive image.)

Coordination of the awarding of outstanding nurse awards and outstanding legislator awards, as well as annual dinners and other events around this day, increases the possibilities for media coverage. Of course someone must be responsible for making the media aware of these events.

Keep in mind that preparations must be made several weeks in advance. Newspapers and radio and television stations must be informed and specific stories suggested. There are special days for all kinds of people—from mothers to secretaries—so the day in itself is not necessarily newsworthy unless you have a story to go with it.

Press releases and radio public-service announcements (PSAs) should be sent out with cover letters persuading the newspaper or station of the importance of their use. Remember to make it clear in your cover letter that airing the PSA is in the public's interest—not just nursing's. (Pointers on developing a

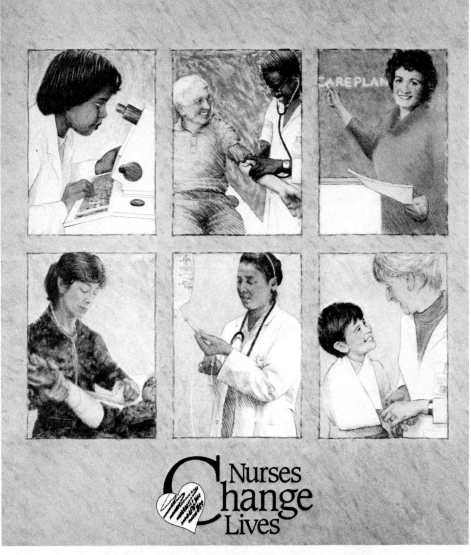

FIG. 5-2. The American Nurses' Association celebrates Nurses' Day 1989. Used with permission of the American Nurses' Association.

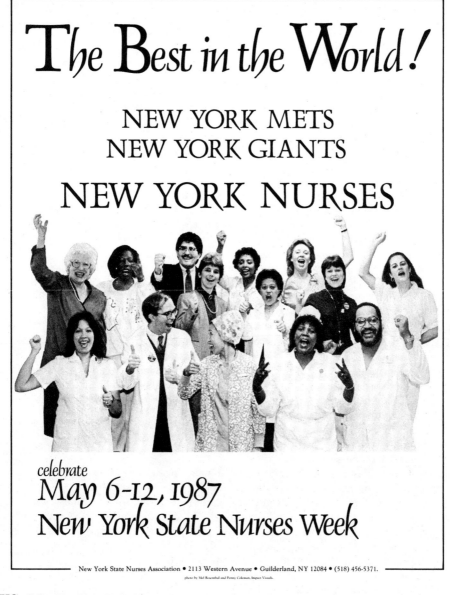

FIG. 5-3. The New York State Nurses Association celebrates Nurses Week 1987. Courtesy New York State Nurses Association.

Format for a Press or Broadcast Release or for a News Story

When preparing a press release or an article, use the following format:
- Type all copy (material written for publication) double spaced on 8½ by 11 inch paper, using one side only.
- Set typewriter for 62 characters to a line. This will ensure 1½ inch margins.
- Give your full name, affiliation, address, phone number, and release date ("For Immediate Release" or "For Release on [a given date]") in the upper, right-hand corner of the first page.
- Begin your story one-third of the way down on the first page.
- Type headline in CAPITAL LETTERS to call the editor's attention to it.
- If release is longer than one page, write "more" at the bottom of each page. Do not break between paragraphs. Instead, break paragraphs in the middle if they fall near the end of the page. This encourages the reader to proceed to the next page.
- For a press release two pages is usually a sufficient length.
- Indicate the end of the release or story by typing pound signs (###) in the center at the bottom of the last page.
- If a photograph or illustration accompanies the story, write "with art" in the bottom, left-hand corner of the last page.
- Hand deliver or address the release to your media contact.
- Be sure the release reaches the publication well before deadline. (Weekly papers may have deadlines a week before publication date.)

VARIATIONS FOR BROADCAST MEDIA RELEASE OR A PUBLIC SERVICE ANNOUNCEMENT

When preparing a release for radio or television, follow the directions given above for formatting a press release. But in addition:
- When writing the copy, think of how it sounds—not how it reads. Such releases can be less formal than those written for newspapers. Use conversational style, and use contractions, such as "don't" instead of "do not." Avoid complicated sentences, and try to pack information into a few words.
- Triple space all copy and type it in all CAPS.
- Submit two copies.
- Never use onion-skin paper.
- Write out all abbreviations, titles, and names. Include the phonetic spellings of unusual names or words in parentheses after correct spelling.
- Be concise. Time the script, count the number of words, then position these numbers prominently on the first page. Radio timing is about 10 seconds for every 25 words. Timing for television should be slightly slower. Public service announcements frequently last 30 seconds.
- To provide more information, also send to the broadcast media the complete release that was sent to newspapers.
- Accompany a PSA with a cover letter telling why airing it is in the public's interest.

**American Nurses' Association
National Nurses' Day 1989
Sample Gubernatorial/Mayoral Proclamation**

Whereas, Nurses have a positive impact on people's lives every day by nature of their keen judgment, compassion, and clinical expertise, and

Whereas, Nurses are the largest group of health care providers in this country, and

Whereas, The demand for nursing services is escalating in light of changes in the financing of health care services, the settings where services are delivered and the health care needs of a graying America, and

Whereas, The supply of nurses is not keeping pace with the demand, and there is an urgent need not only to recruit well-qualified candidates into the profession but to retain nurses in their work environment, and

Whereas, More qualified nurses will be needed in the future to meet the increasingly complex health care needs of the citizens of this state/community, and

Whereas, The American Nurses' Association and the ___(state nurses'___ ___association)___ have declared May 6 as NATIONAL NURSES' DAY 1989 with the theme "Nurses Change Lives" in celebration of the ways in which nurses contribute to high-quality health care and change people's lives, therefore be it

Resolved, That I, ___(Governor's/Mayor's name and title)___ , urge all citizens of this state/community to join me in celebration and recognition of the contributions of nurses and their unique ability to have a positive impact on the lives of those under their care.

---

press release appear in the box on the opposite page. Information regarding development of a PSA can also be found in the box.)

Some state nursing organizations have expanded the one-day observance to Nurses' Week, from May 6 to 12, the last day being Florence Nightingale's birthday. Nurses are encouraged to promote locally the recognition of nursing by the media. Every year enterprising nurses have been the guiding force behind interesting newspaper stories that show nursing at its best.

State and local organizations also arrange for public officials to proclaim National Nurses' Day. A sample proclamation provided by the ANA is seen in the box above. These events provide photo opportunities, which are welcomed by politicians as well as nurses. Arrangements for public presentation of the proclamation must be made well in advance. Governors, county executive officers, and mayors have busy schedules. Contacts must be made with their offices, and an appointment must be made for the ceremony. Someone from the nursing association must be responsible for seeing that the official, nurses, and a photographer are present at the time of the ceremony.

You can assume that it will take at least 2 weeks for the developing and delivery of the photographs. Since you will want the photograph to go with the Nurses' Day story, it is appropriate to schedule the photo session in mid-April.

The public relations committees of many nursing organizations promote celebration of Nurses' Day or Nurses' Week through letters to appropriate hospitals and health agencies. They urge them to plan professional events, suggesting that they invite speakers to discuss health policy or nursing issues instead of following the rather demeaning practice of presenting nurses with flowers or pens. Public recognition of outstanding clinical nurses within the hospital or agency is suggested.

Each year, in anticipation of National Nurses' Day, the ANA provides excellent public relations packets to SNAs in addition to designating a theme. It also makes the packets available to Nurses' Day planners in any professional nursing organization. The kits include guidelines for working with the media, media briefing points, an annotated bibliography, a sample proclamation, a nursing fact sheet, a sample press release, and a camera-ready advertisement.*

WRITING AN ARTICLE

If you are going to write an article or press release yourself, be very clear about your objective. Copy (any material written for publication) that is focused, timely, relevant, and concisely written is more likely to be published. And good photographs or photo possibilities make the material more attractive to editors.

The "lead," or first sentence, must catch the attention of the editor or other readers. It must be dramatic and information-packed, for it may determine whether the release is used.

The "sense" of the story should be given in the first paragraph, answering the questions who, what, when, where, why, and sometimes how.

Be specific. Say something that is informative, not just descriptive. For example, a statement such as "The MNA Legislative Committee met last Saturday" is dull. But "The MNA's Legislative Committee voted to support seat-belt legislation when it met on April 8" provides the reader with vital information.

The inverted pyramid has been used for years to illustrate the structure of a news story (Fig. 5-4). The formula works for press releases also, since they are types of news stories. The first paragraph summarizes the news. Subsequent paragraphs elaborate on and explain the facts in order of decreasing importance. Editors cut from the bottom of a story, if it is necessary to do so, to make the story fit the space available, so the essential story must be told in the first paragraph or two.

---

*To obtain packets for you or your organization, write to the American Nurses' Association, Public Relations Dept., 2420 Pershing Road, Kansas City, MO 64108.

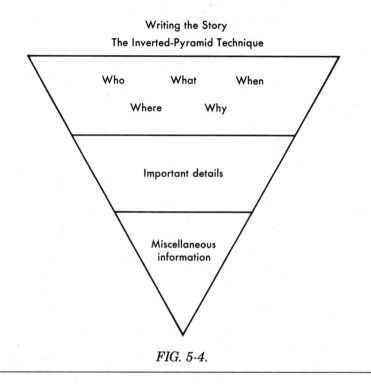

FIG. 5-4.

Here are a few guidelines for effective news writing:
- Use short sentences and paragraphs.
- Use action words, such as "strives," "commands," and "declares."
- Use verbs in the active rather than the passive voice. For example, use "Nurses, spurred on by their leaders, *united* behind the effort to ban smoking in public places" rather than "Nurses *were united* by their leaders behind the effort."
- Write for your audience.
- Avoid clichés and buzz words, particularly the use of nursing jargon. It is practically unintelligible to non-nursing audiences.
- Read and reread copy for errors in spelling, typing, and grammar. Correct them. A second reader is always helpful.
- Sharpen your knowledge of language and style by reviewing references such as William Strunk Jr. and E. B. White's *The Elements of Style;* Kate L. Turabian's *A Manual for Writers of Term Papers, Theses, and Dissertations;* and Theodore M. Bernstein's *The Careful Writer.**

---

*The Elements of Style provides a concise, readable review of English usage, punctuation, and style. *A Manual for Writers of Term Papers, Theses, and Dissertations* is also a useful source of information on style, and *The Careful Writer* is another excellent reference. Other sources are available in bookstores and public libraries.

- At least one style reference, a dictionary, and a thesaurus (which takes its name from a Latin word for "treasure house"—in this case, a treasure house of words) deserve a place near any writer's typewriter.

News releases, whether for print or electronic media, should be prepared in a prescribed format. (See p. 62.) And photos properly used and cared for greatly enhance a story or a presentation. (See box below.)

Guidelines for the Care and Use of Photos

Quality photographs greatly enhance a story. Here are some tips that will help you use them effectively:

- Pictures that tell a story, have some dramatic interest, are best. When possible, plan for them. Show people interacting with each other—not just lined up in a row.
- Politicians and public relations departments of hospitals and health agencies frequently will provide a professional photographer for an event, if one is requested in advance, so be sure to ask. Public relations departments often have "generic" photos, those that represent ideas or concepts, in their files that they are willing to loan. For example, an artful photograph of a visiting nurse carrying her black bag and walking down the street away from the camera could be used to represent community nurses.
- A photo that shows just a person's face, a head shot, is only appropriate if the person is important in the news release.
- For the print media, black-and-white glossy prints are preferred. But whether they are black and white or color prints, they must be well focused and have sharp but not extreme contrast.
- Remember that pictures can and should be cropped (trimmed) by the editor to highlight their best parts.
- Captions should be typed, double spaced, on the lower portion of 8½ by 11 inch paper. They should identify the people in the photo from left to right and should contain the same essential information as the accompanying story's lead. Lower on the paper, identify yourself and your organization and give your address and phone number. Attach the caption to the back of the photo with tape, and fold it over.
- Never write on the back of a photo, especially with ball-point pen. Ink smudges and can damage the clarity of a photo.
- Prepare the photo for mailing by placing it between cardboard inserts. The photo should accompany the press release. Mark the envelope with "Photos—do not bend."

A NEWSLETTER AND HOW IT CAN PROMOTE
AN ASSOCIATION'S LEGISLATIVE PROGRAM

An association's newsletter plays a vital role in promoting both the association and its legislative program. A newsletter filled with relevant information invites readers to become involved in the organization's work.

To be successful, a publication must have a focus. For instance, *The American Nurse* covers the national picture. SNA newsletters, on the other hand, should focus on the people and activities within the state organizations and the nursing issues they are addressing. Because a review of important federal legislative initiatives emphasizes information readers already may have seen in *The American Nurse,* legislative activities at the state capitol should be the primary interest for these publications. District newsletters should concentrate on local programs and the nurses who are active in the district. Since the association is smaller, more informality in writing may be appropriate, for example, use of first names or the title "Ms." with last names rather than last names only after the first reference, as is the accepted style in most print media today. While there may be some overlap of information, if news organizations at each level do their jobs well, they will be more interesting, and nursing will benefit. The same principles apply to any organization that has its own national, state, and local news media.

Good writing, an interesting mix of articles, and an attractive layout that includes good pictures encourage readership. Articles should be written so that any reader can understand what is being said. Almost anyone enjoys seeing her or his name in print: organizations' newsletters should provide that pleasure, as well as recognition for its members. Every association should establish a photo file. Many times a picture can be changed and reused just by cropping it a different way.

An organization's publication is vital to its legislative program. It should educate members about the issues, the legislative process, how they can help, and when that help is needed. (Copies of the publication should also go to the appropriate persons at newspapers and at radio and television stations.)

The *American Journal of Nursing* thinks legislative coverage is so important that when it presents awards for excellence to SNA publications, it has a special category for such coverage. I was asked to judge the 1987 entries. As I went through them, I looked for news publications that demonstrated a consistent focus on legislative issues, explained them clearly, and showed nurses how to use their influence in the politics of health care.

In the three winning entries—*The Minnesota Nurses Association Accent* (or *MNA Accent*), *The Kansas Nurse,* and *South Dakota Nurse*—both state and federal legislative issues were covered thoroughly. The bill-by-bill synopses of proposed legislation relevant to nursing were clear and were complete enough to convey the bills' contents understandably.

The entire January 1987 issue of *The Kansas Nurse* focused on the "Nurse as Politician" (Fig. 5-5). It included five major articles, each with a different focus on the relevance of nurses' involvement in politics:

> "A Vehicle for Political Socialization," an article by Barbara E. Langner, RN, PhD, and Susan H. Fetsch, RN, MS, described an elective course for undergraduate nursing students called "Political Strategies for Health Care Professionals," aimed

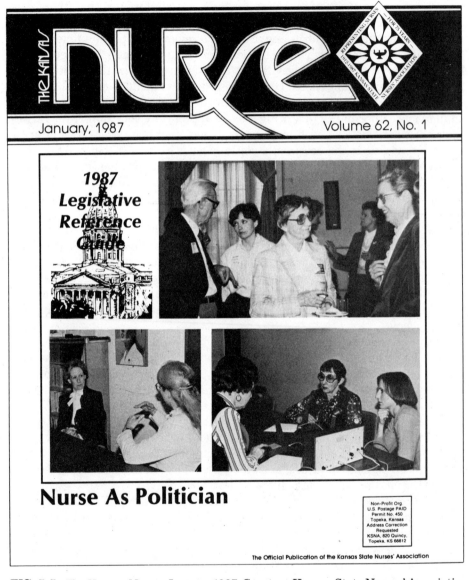

FIG. 5-5. The Kansas Nurse, January 1987. Courtesy Kansas State Nurses' Association.

at promoting understanding of the political process and its effect on nursing practice.[2]

Judy Runnels, a nurse and at the time a candidate for Secretary of State in Kansas, described her interest in politics in an interview with Susan Tannenwald-Miringoff, RN, JD, in "Reflections of a Political Nurse."[3]

Senator Roy Ehrlich, Chairman of the Kansas Senate's Public Health and Welfare Committee, provided a preview of the 1987 Kansas legislative session in an interview titled "We Must Live Within Our Means."[4]

An extensive "1987 Legislative Toolchest" included the legislative platform of the Kansas State Nurses' Association (KSNA), important phone numbers, resources for learning about legislation, information on how to write to legislators, a review of KSNA legislative activities, lists of the names and phone numbers of Kansas state senators and representatives, U.S. senators and representatives, people in leadership positions in the House and the Senate, and KSNA district legislative chairpersons, maps of the state of Kansas showing legislative-district boundaries, and a graphic showing how a bill becomes a law.[5]

Nickie Stein, RN, MEd, 1987 KSNA legislative chairperson, wrote a legislative update: "Lobbying for Better Health Care: A 'Natural' for a Nurse."[6]

Finally, the issue included a promotion for the KSNA's upcoming Day at the Legislature. (A sample of the registration form for the 1989 program is shown in Fig. 5-6.) This issue of *The Kansas Nurse* represented comprehensive, educational coverage of legislation and legislative activities and worthily received commendation.

All three of the award-winning publications had clearly delineated legislative sections that were designed to hold the reader's attention. *South Dakota Nurse* highlighted its legislative section by printing it on colored paper. The *MNA Accent* included thumbnail photos of sponsoring legislators with its description of bills given high priority by the MNA.

Many nursing organizations send their publications to legislators, at least during the legislative session. Feature articles about nurses in different kinds of practice settings promote nursing's image and reduce the mystery surrounding nurses' jobs. Occasional short profiles about legislators who support nursing are another way of reinforcing good relationships. Be sure to include photographs, which can be obtained by calling legislators' offices.

Nurses who are legislators or candidates for office must be promoted. Nursing publications must regularly cover the news generated by the activities of nurses who have just been elected to office and those already holding office, but this coverage is even more important during election years. In addition, publications can promote new candidates by introducing them to readers through stories about their activities and feature stories and by encouraging them to write for the publication.

Announcements must be made of nursing PACs' endorsements of candidates seeking offices at both the state and federal levels, and follow-up stories must be written. National stories should be localized. For example, ANA/PAC gave a high-priority endorsement to Barbara Mikulski's successful candidacy for the U.S. Senate in 1986. *The Maryland Nurse*'s story on the endorsement included comments by Maryland nurses.

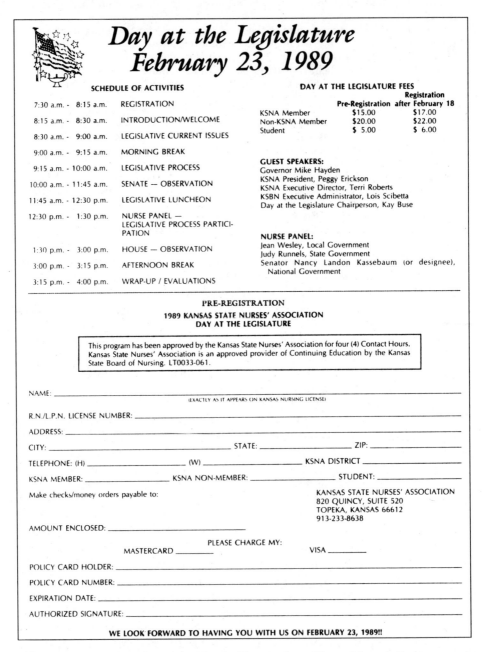

Day at the Legislature
February 23, 1989

SCHEDULE OF ACTIVITIES

7:30 a.m. - 8:15 a.m.	REGISTRATION
8:15 a.m. - 8:30 a.m.	INTRODUCTION/WELCOME
8:30 a.m. - 9:00 a.m.	LEGISLATIVE CURRENT ISSUES
9:00 a.m. - 9:15 a.m.	MORNING BREAK
9:15 a.m. - 10:00 a.m.	LEGISLATIVE PROCESS
10:00 a.m. - 11:45 a.m.	SENATE — OBSERVATION
11:45 a.m. - 12:30 p.m.	LEGISLATIVE LUNCHEON
12:30 p.m. - 1:30 p.m.	NURSE PANEL — LEGISLATIVE PROCESS PARTICIPATION
1:30 p.m. - 3:00 p.m.	HOUSE — OBSERVATION
3:00 p.m. - 3:15 p.m.	AFTERNOON BREAK
3:15 p.m. - 4:00 p.m.	WRAP-UP / EVALUATIONS

DAY AT THE LEGISLATURE FEES

	Pre-Registration	Registration after February 18
KSNA Member	$15.00	$17.00
Non-KSNA Member	$20.00	$22.00
Student	$ 5.00	$ 6.00

GUEST SPEAKERS:
Governor Mike Hayden
KSNA President, Peggy Erickson
KSNA Executive Director, Terri Roberts
KSBN Executive Administrator, Lois Scibetta
Day at the Legislature Chairperson, Kay Buse

NURSE PANEL:
Jean Wesley, Local Government
Judy Runnels, State Government
Senator Nancy Landon Kassebaum (or designee), National Government

PRE-REGISTRATION
1989 KANSAS STATE NURSES' ASSOCIATION
DAY AT THE LEGISLATURE

> This program has been approved by the Kansas State Nurses' Association for four (4) Contact Hours. Kansas State Nurses' Association is an approved provider of Continuing Education by the Kansas State Board of Nursing. LT0033-061.

NAME: _____
(EXACTLY AS IT APPEARS ON KANSAS NURSING LICENSE)

R.N./L.P.N. LICENSE NUMBER: _____

ADDRESS: _____

CITY: _____ STATE: _____ ZIP: _____

TELEPHONE: (H) _____ (W) _____ KSNA DISTRICT _____

KSNA MEMBER: _____ KSNA NON-MEMBER: _____ STUDENT: _____

Make checks/money orders payable to: KANSAS STATE NURSES' ASSOCIATION
820 QUINCY, SUITE 520
TOPEKA, KANSAS 66612
913-233-8638

AMOUNT ENCLOSED: _____

PLEASE CHARGE MY:

MASTERCARD _____   VISA _____

POLICY CARD HOLDER: _____

POLICY CARD NUMBER: _____

EXPIRATION DATE: _____

AUTHORIZED SIGNATURE: _____

WE LOOK FORWARD TO HAVING YOU WITH US ON FEBRUARY 23, 1989!!

FIG. 5-6. Attractive publicity used by the Kansas State Nurses' Association to promote their "Day at the Legislature, February 23, 1989." Note the program and the registration form are both on one page. (Reprinted by permission from the Kansas State Nurses' Association.)

Relevant, readable, and attractive newsletters are vital to nursing's future effectiveness in legislation and politics.

CORRECTING AND EXPANDING THE RECORD

Many of us have reacted in anger to what we consider inaccurate representations of nurses and nursing in both the print and electronic media. There are times when we must respond either to correct the record or to expand on information that is inadequate as presented. We can respond individually or collectively. As so often occurs in political situations, numbers count. Media representatives are more likely to respond to group pressure—but sometimes that pressure must be maintained for some time.

Television

One of the outstanding victories in defense of nursing's media image is in the script changes in later *M*A*S*H* episodes that made the character of Major Margaret Houlihan more acceptable to nurses. In early episodes of this long-running television series, Margaret was appropriately nicknamed "Hot Lips." In later episodes, while her basic character remained intact, she was no longer represented as promiscuous. These changes were a result of continued pressure from nurses and their organizations to improve Margaret's image as it reflected on nursing. Actor Alan Alda, star of the series, who has a reputation for sensitivity to women's issues, is credited with giving nurses' complaints a sympathetic ear.

In 1989 the NBC television network launched *Nightingales,* a prime-time television series that focused on the lives of a group of nursing students. The nursing community was less than pleased. While some episodes attempted in an awkward way to deal with real nursing issues, such scenes were overshadowed by those that showed off the physical attributes of the female students—frequently shown scantily clad in showers and locker rooms.

Story lines were also objectionable. One regular in the series, though reformed, had a history of drug and alcohol dependence. In one episode another student's boyfriend overdosed on drugs and died, so the student was accused (though falsely) of having supplied him with the fatal drugs.

The nursing community reacted in horror. The ANA had received hundreds of complaints about the pilot, which had aired earlier in the year, and had attempted to use its muscle with the network to derail the program, but to no avail. While the series was somewhat toned down, nurses felt even more outraged that a major network would initiate a series so damaging to nursing's image at a time when the Secretary's Commission on Nursing was citing negative image as an important cause of the nursing shortage.

On February 7, 1989, The *Washington Post*'s health section carried a cover story titled "If Florence Nightingale Could See Them Now: TV Image of Nurses

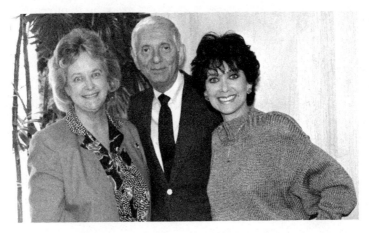

Left to right: Dr. Lucille Joel, President of the ANA, Aaron Spelling, producer of *Nightingales,* and Suzanne Pleshette, star of the series. From The American Nurse, May 1989, p. 4.

Hits New Low, and Real Nurses are Up in Arms."[7] The story attracted a flood of letters to the editor reacting negatively to *Nightingales* and appreciatively to the *Post* for publishing the article.

Nursing associations quickly organized to get the series off the air. Organizational newsletters published the name and address of the president of NBC, as well as those of the producers of the series and the presidents of the program's commercial sponsors. They encouraged nurses to write these people to protest the program's representation of nursing, to tell them how injurious the show was to professional nursing, and to advise sponsors that they would boycott their products as long as they continued to advertise on *Nightingales*.

NBC did not renew the series for the fall season. While general campaigns to clean up television were at least partly responsible for the show's demise, much of the credit for getting *Nightingales* off the air went to professional nursing associations for the pressure they exerted. Aaron Spelling, the show's executive producer, was quoted in the *Washington Post* in June 1989 as saying, "I don't think there's any doubt in the world that if we hadn't had that nurses thing, we would have been picked up (for the fall season)."[8]

The cancellation of the series proved that when committed and organized to work for a common goal, nurses can be enormously effective. This cancellation is an excellent example of a situation in which nurses actively defended their image and won.

---

*Joel met with Spelling to discuss nursing's concerns about the show. She shared ideas for story lines that would portray the realities of nursing practice. After the meeting, Joel said, "I heard a commitment that if 'Nightingales' is renewed for the fall 1989 TV season, it will portray nursing accurately and positively."[9]

I enjoyed Abigail Trafford's commentary, "If Florence Nightingale Could See Them Now" (Cover Story, Feb. 7). Poor Flo must be spinning in her grave on Wednesday evenings when NBC's "Corps des Bimbettes" makes its appearance on "Nightingales." The only nursing stereotypes not explored in depth by this show are the ones related to caring, competence and compassion.

America has an undeniable nursing crisis that is in part the result of two decades of steadily deteriorating media portrayals of the profession. Wouldn't it be wonderful to once again see a show that casts a strong, intelligent, witty individual in a nursing role, and backed up that actor or actress with week after week of finely crafted script material? Fortunately, one does not have to rely on reruns of "St. Elsewhere" for this . . . just flip the dial to ABC and be treated to Dana Delaney's exquisite performance on "China Beach." Her unforgettable character, McMurphy, may single-handedly rejuvenate the image of the nursing profession.

Jim Walters
Silver Spring

We of the Navy Nurse Corps experience many of the same challenges as our civilian counterparts in trying to attract the best nursing talent. A positive, accurate image of nursing is vital to the health of military nursing.

Professional nursing organizations are increasing their efforts to show the public the realities of nursing—the important role nurses play, their high level of education and training, and the degree of professionalism and dedication found in both the civilian and military nurse communities. Your article goes a long way toward achieving that goal.

Mary F. Hall
Rear Admiral, Nurse Corps, USN
Director, Navy Nurse Corps
Washington

The article captured the essence of the difficulties the nursing profession has faced and fought these past few years. We aren't sitting still and allowing this assault on our profession to take place quietly. The Montgomery County Chapter of the Maryland Nurses' Association sent a letter to NBC that expresses our strong opposition to a program that personifies every myth and stereotype ever conceived regarding the nursing profession.

The public needs to know that nurses are caring, dedicated, responsible professionals who are required to work under many adverse conditions, one of those being an unfair and inaccurate perception of what nursing is, largely because of media portrayals such as that in "Nightingales." We won't be satisfied until that program is removed from the air.

Patrice Robins, BSN, RN
Executive Board Member
Montgomery County Chapter
Maryland Nurses' Association
Rockville

Thank goodness someone has the courage to tell the truth about the blasphemy presented on the TV program "The Nightingales." The producers of this scurrilous program need to visit intensive care wards in clinical care units with patients with AIDS to see how "real" professional nurses function. God forbid if the producers have to have a coronary (which they deserve) to learn about real nursing.

Nursing for the past century has been a proud and noble profession—one that can be a rewarding career for both men and women.

Rear Adm. Faye G. Abdellah
Deputy Surgeon General
U.S. Public Health Service

From *The Washington Post*, February 21, 1989.

Letters to the Editor

To the Editor:

Your letters in "Nurse Shortage is Not Sudden or Surprising" (July 18) were disturbing to me and my colleagues but certainly not surprising, as they are typical of some of the misperceptions that cling to nursing.

Indeed, salaries have not advanced as rapidly as the responsibilities of the "bedside" nurse. However, Frank H. Scarangella (husband of a nurse) is grossly uninformed about what the American Nurses Association has done to raise salaries. The association's division of economic and general welfare, established in 1946, organized nurses all over the country and now bargains for more nurses than any other group. It is through its efforts that nursing salaries have achieved today's levels. Starting salaries in New York City, for example, are now $26,000 to $32,000. It is even more painful that Mr. Scarangella is married to a nursing educator, because it is the Nursing Association that won equal pension rights for nursing faculty members. Moreover, it was because of the association's lobbying that stipends for higher education were awarded.

As for "A National Service Job?", Clinton G. Weiman's implication is clear and echoes the sentiments of many old-guard physicians: anyone, especially a female, can do a nurse's job. Dr. Weiman's suggestion that all 17- and 18-year-olds be drafted to work in hospitals is astonishing, when one considers that professional nurse education requires two to four years academic preparation and at least a year of practice before a new graduate feels competent to juggle the technology, the ever-changing treatments and drugs, and be a source of solace and support, as well as an advocate for patients who are sicker than ever before. Adding more rank beginners to such a high-tech environment is harking back to a simpler past that no longer exists.

Finally, Dr. Alan D. Lieberson's view that nursing school enrollments are plummeting because of acquired immune deficiency syndrome is far too simplistic. Nursing has faced, head on, the influenza outbreaks of World War I, the tuberculosis outbreaks of the 1930's and the polio epidemics of the 50's. Nursing has never been "safe." Yet today, nurses are not only volunteering, but they are even lining up to work in AIDS units.

Nancy A. Moree
New York, July 22, 1987

The writer, a registered nurse, is director of medical nursing at Presbyterian Hospital.

OPEN THE DOOR TO COLLEGE AS AN INCENTIVE
FOR WOULD-BE NURSES

To the Editor:

While I applaud "This Nursing Shortage Is Different" (editorial, Dec. 20) and the recommendations of the Federal commission on nursing, as a public official concerned about the level of health care offered our citizens, and as a former nurse, I feel much more is needed.

While the commission's recommendations on increasing salaries, resuming student loans, offering flexible work schedules and eliminating non-nursing tasks will help address the nursing shortage, we must also take immediate action to attract more people into nursing in the first place and then encourage them to remain professional nurses in hospital service.

One effective measure to achieve this would be enactment of the nursing shortage relief bill, which I helped develop with Representative Gary L. Ackerman of Queens, and which he introduced in Congress.

Through a series of scholarships, loan forgivenesses and other incentives, our nation would enable young people interested in professional nursing to obtain a college education. We would open the door to college to many who could not otherwise obtain higher education.

The idea for this program came from my own experience. During World War II, our nation faced a nursing crisis similar in magnitude to the one we are confronted with today. Many nurses left hospitals for the military, and most nursing school graduates were going directly into the armed services. Congress passed the Bolten Act, and I received free tuition, board, books, uniforms and a small stipend to major in nursing at college. This same type of assistance and encouragement is needed today.

In addition, the act would provide funds to hospitals and colleges to recruit potential students and encourage nonpracticing nurses to return to nursing. Other provisions would make nursing more attractive by providing career advancement, make nurses a more integral part of hospital operations and increase the prestige and recognition of nurses.

The bill will be reintroduced in next year's Congress. Its speedy consideration and enactment will be a major weapon in meeting the nursing crisis that you, the nursing commission and others have recognized.

It also will go a long way to assuring that our nation will have a key element in its health delivery program—an adequate pool of well-trained, properly motivated, career professional nurses.

Claire Shulman
Queens Borough President
Kew Gardens, Queens, Dec. 23, 1988

Letters to the Editor

Well-written letters to the editor may be the most effective way that nurses, as individuals or through their associations, can correct misinformation, expand on issues raised in previously published news or feature stories, or thank editors for their coverage of an issue.

The examples on p. 73 show how nurses in Washington, D.C., responded to the *Washington Post* article regarding *Nightingales*.

Another example of an effective letter to the editor appeared in the August 10, 1987, issue of the *New York Times* (see box on p. 74). Nancy A. Moree responded to an article about the nursing shortage that had appeared in the *Times*. Moree, director of medical nursing at New York's Presbyterian Hospital, challenged the opinions of several people who had been quoted in the article and strongly defended nursing's dedication to professionalism and patient care. The letter was more than a complaint: the writer offered relevant new information.

In still another example from the *New York Times,* the writer recommends one avenue for the alleviation of the nursing shortage. (Note that the letter's author, Claire Shulman, is president of the Borough of Queens, one of five jurisdictions that make up New York City.) Using her nursing background and her influence, Shulman worked with the U.S. congressman from her district to develop a bill to provide scholarship funds for student nurses. The letter also illustrates the advantage to the nursing profession of having nurses in public office.

Issues more substantive than the example which follows are more deserving of letters or opinion pieces in the print media. But this example highlights the practical points to be considered in getting such a letter published.

In March 1987 Russell Myers, creator of the popular comic strip "Broom Hilda," did a series of frames portraying the little witch as a nurse (Fig. 5-7). While the series was meant to be comic, it was damaging to nursing's image. Other frames were demeaning also, but those in Fig. 5-7 illustrate the point. The first frame showed nursing as menial; the second implied that nurses don't care about errors involving medication.

Writing Effective Letters to the Editor

In constructing a letter to the editor, summarize the issue to which you are reacting. Make your response, and then present information to back up your opinion. Facts and figures strengthen your case. Such responses must be prompt—newspapers emphasize timeliness. Note that the cartoon in question appeared on March 3, the letter was mailed on March 4, and the response was published on March 7. Of course, editors have to choose among the different letters they receive, so a well-presented case and relevance are important. Some newspapers will telephone you to confirm that you wrote the letter before pub-

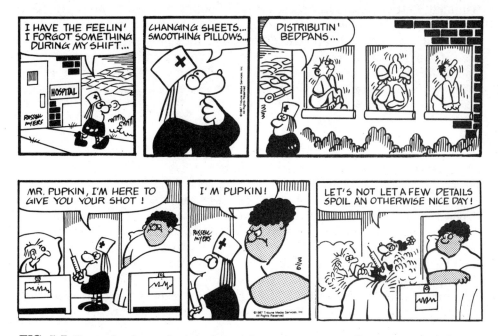

FIG. 5-7. Example of a comic strip demeaning to nurses, as well as a prompt, informative response. Reprinted by permission: Tribune Media Services.

Letter to the Editor

To the Editor:

The "Broom Hilda" cartoon that appeared on March 3 was not only tasteless; it was also insulting to the nation's 1.5 million registered nurses. The whole series is demeaning, but this installment implied that nursing's focus is "changing sheets, smoothing pillows, and distributin' bedpans."

Cartoonist Russell Myers should know that today's nurses practicing in hospitals are responsible for around-the-clock professional observation, care involving sophisticated technology and comprehensive health teaching of patients.

In addition, registered nurses provide needed services in the community—in patients' homes, health maintenance organizations, nursing homes, free-standing surgical facilities, schools, clinics, industry, psychiatric institutions and centers for the aging. Nationally, more than 20,000 nurses are in advanced independent practice.

Members of the nursing profession deserve recognition for their vital contributions to the nation's health—not the kind of message projected by Myers' cartoon.

Mary Lloyd Zusy, R.N.

lishing it. Letters should be addressed to the editor of the editorial page. His or her name and the address of the newspaper can be found on the newspaper's masthead, which usually appears on the editorial page.

If you can become recognized by the media as a credible source on nursing and health care issues, you can be immensely influential. But for day-to-day media exposure, letters to the editor are probably the most effective way to get your point of view into the print media.

Advertisers

Advertisers are sensitive to negative comment; moreover, they thrive on the positive reception of their material by the public. Letters and phone calls responding to negative nursing images should be sent directly to them or to the general managers of local television stations and editors of local newspapers.

One such case involved a Baltimore health maintenance organization (HMO), which used a picture of a witch-like nurse to dramatize the care clients might receive at other HMOs. The publicity committee of the Maryland Nurses' Association responded immediately with strong letters of protest to both the HMO and the television station. The MNA's prompt response brought an apology from the advertiser, and the offensive ad was taken off the air.

PREPARATION FOR A RADIO OR TELEVISION INTERVIEW

We must seek opportunities for articulate, well-informed nurses to represent nursing before the large audiences commanded by radio and television.

Whether or not formal speakers' bureaus are established, it is up to nursing organizations to promote nurses' appearances on interview programs on radio and television. Someone—either the chairperson of the speakers' bureau or a member of the public relations committee—must notify stations that nursing experts are available to speak on health issues. This is done most easily by sending letters to station managers. Reminders must then be made by telephone when nursing or health-policy issues arise in which we have an interest.

Frequently, nurses are finding themselves being interviewed on television and radio in connection with breaking news stories. Whether the interview is informal and spur-of-the-moment or carefully orchestrated, you will need to keep the same things in mind:

Always be prepared. Be knowledgeable about the subject under discussion. Have relevant facts in mind. Try to anticipate the questions you are likely to be asked, and know how you will word your answers. If possible, rehearse with a friend who will give you constructive criticism.

Make your points briefly and clearly and in language the interviewer and the audience will understand. Avoid long-winded explanations. Help the inter-

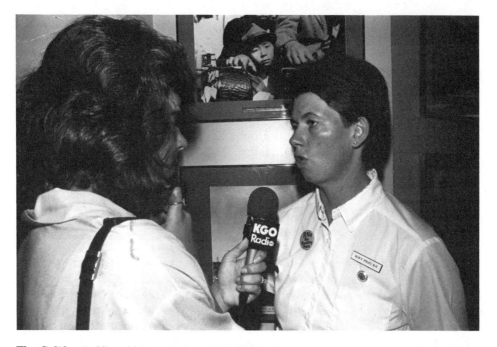

The California Nurses' Association's Mary Foley responds to a radio reporter's questions about the nursing shortage. (From *The California Nurse,* photographer Marjorie McCloy.)

viewer know what you think is important by saying something like, "The important point is. . . ." Try to keep the interview focused on your message.

Kalisch and Kalisch[10] urge nurses to be active advocates rather than passive respondents in interview situations. They suggest that when presented with irrelevant questions and/or loaded prefaces, you answer the question briefly and form a bridge to your idea of what is important. We think a young woman in our community did it well when, in a recent television interview regarding the nursing shortage, she was asked, "Don't you think that if there were more men in nursing, your problems would be solved?" She responded:

> We believe that it would be valuable to have more men in nursing, but the male/female ratio is not really relevant to the nursing shortage. What is needed is better working conditions for nurses, increased salaries, more scholarship funds for nursing education, and more public recognition for nursing's vital contributions to the nation's health care.

As in other situations, your appearance counts, so dress appropriately for interviews. Solid colors—medium tones of blue, gray, or brown—work best for television. Whether sitting or standing, keep your posture erect. Try to project an image of confident professionalism.

NURSES AS TELEVISION PRODUCERS AND HEALTH COLUMNISTS

Some nurses have stepped into positions as television producers and health columnists. One such person is Madeline Turkeltaub, RN, PhD, director of the nursing program at Montgomery Community College in Takoma Park, Maryland. She is the producer of a half-hour interview program called *Healthier Living*. Produced at Montgomery College, the program is shown on both the campus and the Montgomery County cable channels. Every show is aired four times in two weeks on each channel.

It began when Turkeltaub approached the people organizing a cable television station within the college. She had had some experience producing educational videos and looked on the station as a golden opportunity. Organizers were looking for program material, and Turkeltaub was able to present a strong, credible proposal. She persuaded organizers that it would be appropriate for a registered nurse to produce a program featuring general information on health. At the time, a county cable television station was also being organized, and it picked up *Healthier Living*. At this writing, a Virginia cable station is interested in her show.

Turkeltaub introduces herself by saying, "I'm Dr. Madeline Turkeltaub. I am a registered nurse and the director of the nursing program at Montgomery College." She believes her introduction gives the public two important pieces of positive information about nursing: that some nurses have advanced degrees and that some nurses also head departments in institutions of higher learning. And the quality of the program shows that nurses are interested in and knowledgeable about substantive health care issues.

In the program, Turkeltaub tries to be a patient advocate. She seeks answers to the kinds of questions patients would ask. The program is very practical. For instance, when she hosted a show urging cigarette smokers to give up the habit, three of her four panelists were former smokers who could answer questions from their own experience. On another show, Turkeltaub featured representatives from the Washington Transplant Consortium, who appealed for organ donors. When she ran a series of programs on how legislation affects health care, she asked me to interview our county executive during one show and U.S. Senator Barbara Mikulski during another program.

Instead of commercial breaks, Turkeltaub features one-minute segments called "health breaks," which are run like advertisements. One features exercises people can do sitting in a chair—a help for the chair-bound viewer—and another gives tips on diet.

Turkeltaub invites members of the nursing community to suggest program topics. The program provides a public service, as well as a fine public relations opportunity for nursing. Producing such a television program is something that articulate, well-informed nurses with some technical experience could do anywhere.[11]

Some nurses write health columns for their local newspapers. To be considered as a television producer or newspaper columnist, you must approach the appropriate management person in either the print or electronic media with a strong proposal, your résumé, and a few samples of the product you propose. A regular program or column requires a substantial commitment of time, energy, and ideas. But the personal rewards are great, and the benefit to nursing is substantial.

GETTING OUR MESSAGE ACROSS

Persuasion is indispensable to the art of politics. As individuals we can make a difference, through studying the issues, drawing conclusions, and presenting our points of view so effectively that we persuade others to support us in the public arena. We can improve our own and nursing's image. Involvement in community groups and grass-roots politics is one way to educate the public about nursing. But if we can learn to work effectively with representatives from newspapers, radio, and television, our opportunities to influence will be greatly expanded. We must persuade media representatives of our professionalism and nursing's vital interest in health policy. We must lead them to stories that exemplify these nursing attributes. Often, responding to an unfavorable representation of nursing may be an effective way to correct the record and improve the profession's image.

We must continue to improve our organizational publications, making them meaningful and informative. Publications must promote the association's legislative agenda in a practical way by showing members why they should become involved and how they can help. And we must put media representatives who may be interested in our initiatives on the mailing list.

Most nursing organizations cannot support paid professionals to manage public relations; therefore, each of us is responsible for doing her or his part. Basically, public relations is every nurse's business. We must heighten our awareness of opinion-molding possibilities and work together to make a positive difference in the public's perceptions of nursing.

REFERENCES

1. Kalisch BJ and Kalisch PA: Communicating clinical nursing issues through the newspaper, Nursing Research 30(3):132-138, 1981.
2. Langner BE and Fetsch SH: A vehicle for political socialization, The Kansas Nurse (62)1:1, 1987.
3. Tannenwald-Miringoff S: Reflections of a political nurse, The Kansas Nurse 62(1):3, 1987.

4. Ehrlich R: We must live within our means, The Kansas Nurse 62(1):6, 1987.
5. Stein N and Tannenwald-Miringoff S: 1987 legislative toolchest, The Kansas Nurse 62(1):7-17, 1987.
6. Stein N: Lobbying for better health care: a "Natural" for a nurse, The Kansas Nurse 62(1):16, 1987.
7. Tafford A: If Florence Nightingale could see them now: TV image of nurses hits new low, and real nurses are up in arms, Washington Post, p H12, February 7, 1989.
8. Shales T: Attack of the TV reformers: the aftermath of a salty season, Washington Post, p G1, June 25, 1989.
9. Grimaldi C: Joel meets with producer of *Nightingales* series, The American Nurse 21(5):4, 1989.
10. Kalisch BJ and Kalisch PA: Good news, bad news, or no news: improving radio and TV coverage of nursing issues, Nursing and Health Care 6(5):255-260, 1985.
11. Turkeltaub M: Personal communication, March 1989.

Chapter **6**

THE LEGISLATIVE PROCESS: FROM CONCEPTION TO IMPLEMENTATION OF A LAW

If we nurses are to use legislation to benefit the public, ourselves, and our profession, we must understand not only legislative procedures, but also how to make them work. In this chapter we will talk about the legislative process. We will describe how Maryland nurses influenced it to pioneer legislation that requires insurance companies to compensate directly nurse-midwives, nurse-practitioners, and nurse-anesthetists in independent practice for health care services they are licensed to provide.

This action by Maryland nurses illustrates the rewards of working in state legislatures for professional nursing's goals. Indeed these goals are many and the means to their achievement accessible. First, both the state capitol and state legislators are within our reach. The state capitol can be no more than a few hours' drive for any nurse, and it is easier to pass legislation there than in the U.S. Congress, because in any one state, there is less diversity and, consequently, less controversy. State legislators are more accessible to their constituents than are their federal counterparts, not only because many of their interests are local but also because they have more time and smaller staffs. At this level there are real opportunities for us as individuals and in organized nursing groups to influence the legislative process.

Furthermore, the work done in one state legislature frequently influences events beyond the state line. Once a precedent is set, it provides a workable model for other state legislatures. Inspired by Maryland nurses' success in getting third-party reimbursement for nurses in advanced practice, nurses in other parts of the country have pushed for similar legislation in their states, and many have been successful.

Finally, experience gained in making legislation work at the state level frequently helps shape an effective and workable federal policy. In recent years Congress has mandated reimbursement to nurse-midwives for some services under Medicaid and Medicare. In 1978 Congress passed legislation requiring direct reimbursement of certified nurse-midwives in independent practice for services they provide to dependents of active-duty personnel and eligible retirees insured under the Department of Defense Civilian Health and Medical Program of the Uniformed Services (CHAMPUS). In 1981 Congress followed up by including direct reimbursement to nurse-practitioners as part of CHAMPUS coverage.

All of the 400 fee-for-service insurance plans offered in the Federal Employee Health Benefit Program (FEHBP), with the exception of one in the Panama Canal zone, cover the services of nurse-midwives. Presently efforts are being made to broaden FEHBP policies to include direct reimbursement of nurse-practitioners and nurse-anesthetists. If passed, this legislation would further expand opportunities for nurses in independent practice. Approximately 8.8 million federal employees, annuitants, and dependents are covered by FEHBP.[1]

Whether nurses work at the state or federal level, knowledge of the legislative process is essential. But before we discuss the process of how a bill becomes law, let's review some of the basics of how the U.S. government works. In establishing the U.S. Constitution, our country's founders worked diligently to find mechanisms by which the needs of the people could be met, the rights of minorities protected, and conflicting interests reconciled. The system of checks and balances they established was adopted by framers of state constitutions, who modeled them on the federal system, with minor variations. Let's first talk briefly about the federal system.

THE FEDERAL GOVERNMENT

The executive branch of government implements laws. In the federal government the president is the chief executive. The president provides leadership, promotes public policy and lobbies for legislation that will make it law, and conducts foreign policy.

The legislative branch consists of the U.S. Congress, a bicameral (or two-house) body that enacts laws, often after receiving input from a variety of sources. Congress has specific authority over most federal spending, except certain programs financed by special trust funds, such as Social Security.

Newly enacted laws are, in effect, only authorizations for programs. For them to be implemented, Congress must pass appropriations, or spending, bills, all of which are initiated in the House of Representatives. To keep the government operating and existing programs funded, Congress must pass annual appropriations bills. This control over the purse strings of the federal government gives Congress a powerful lever for influencing the direction of national policy. And it provides an effective system of checks and balances between the legislative and executive branches of government.

In addition to dealing with legislative matters, the U.S. Senate, the upper house, confirms or rejects certain presidential appointments, including nominees to the Supreme Court and ambassadors. Membership in the 100-member Senate is based on equal representation for each state. For example, sparsely populated Alaska has the same number of representatives (two) in the Senate as does densely populated New York. A U.S. senator's term of office lasts 6 years. In the Senate, terms are staggered, so that approximately one third of its members are up for election every 2 years.

The number of representatives to the lower house, or House of Representatives, is apportioned among the states according to population, with each member representing a specified number of voters. In 1989, there were 435 members in the House. They are titled "representative," or "congressman," or "congresswoman." Their terms of office last 2 years.

The most powerful official in Congress is the speaker of the House, elected by the members of the majority party in the House of Representatives. The speaker is the presiding officer of the chamber. He conducts the House's business, handles scheduling of legislation for floor action, interprets rules, refers bills to committees, and appoints members of the select and conference committees.

The Senate's most powerful member is the majority leader, who, like the speaker of the House, is elected by the members of the majority party in that chamber. The vice-president of the United States is the presiding officer of the Senate.

Both houses of Congress are organized along party lines—Democratic and Republican. The majority leader in each house speaks for the party in power. The minority leader organizes the party's work and serves as its official spokesperson. The minority leader's duties correspond to those of the majority leader, except that he or she has no authority over the scheduling of legislation. Each party also appoints a "whip" to assist the leader in organizing support for the party's legislative program.

Essentially all of Congress' work is done in standing and ad hoc committees. Chairpersons are elected by committee members of the majority party, but precedent dictates that these important positions usually go to the party's senior member. Committees and individual legislators also have staffs that assist them in their work. Interest in a particular piece of legislation by the committee chairperson, committee members, and staff members is essential to its passage. Therefore, anyone hoping to influence the outcome of a legislative initiative must know the name of the committee to which a bill has been assigned and the names of the committee's chairperson and members. This information can be obtained by writing or telephoning your legislator. The American Nurses' Association's Washington office* or the Washington headquarters of other national nursing organizations can provide this information about health care and nursing bills.

---

*1101 14th St, NW, Suite 200, Washington, D.C. 20005.

In their wisdom the authors of the U.S. Constitution provided mechanisms intended to ensure proper study and debate, as well as a measure of consensus, before a bill can become law. During the 1988 legislative session, 11,282 bills were introduced in Congress. Of that number, 713 became laws. In state legislatures the ratio of bills introduced to laws enacted is similar. Only a fraction of those proposed actually become law.

Legislation may be reintroduced repeatedly in either Congress or the state legislatures. Acceptance of new ideas takes time. To build a consensus, work must be done within the legislature and outside its chambers. Such was the case, you may remember, in the effort to gain women's suffrage. Legislation was introduced, reintroduced, and regularly debated for more than 40 years before a consensus was reached and a constitutional amendment incorporated into the laws of the land.

Part of the function of the judicial system is to interpret laws that are challenged by individuals or groups. Such challenges are initiated in the lower courts. Through the appeals process, cases may be reviewed repeatedly until they reach the Supreme Court, the highest court in the United States. Decisions made by the courts influence how laws are implemented. Anyone who has watched a television show or movie with the police in it is acquainted with an obvious example: in 1966 a Supreme Court decision in the *Miranda v. Arizona* case set a precedent requiring all law officers to advise people of their constitutional rights at the time of arrest. These rights include the right to remain silent, the right to be informed that anything they say can be used again them in a court of law, and the right to have a lawyer present during questioning.

STATE GOVERNMENTS

Most state constitutions parallel the federal system, but there are some differences. The governor is the chief executive in state government. State legislatures may also be called general or legislative assemblies. (In New Hampshire the legislature is called the General Court.) Most state legislatures, like the federal model, are bicameral. (Nebraska's legislature, however, is unicameral, and members of its one chamber are called senators.) Members of the lower houses in different states may be called representatives, delegates, or assemblymen or assemblywomen. Terms of office for both state senators and representatives vary from state to state.

Most state legislatures have the authority to develop their own budgets. However, there are a few states in which an executive budget system limits legislative input. As in Congress, much of the work of state legislatures is done in committees. Nurses interested in promoting their legislative programs must know which committees deal with nursing and health policy legislation, as well as the names of their chairpersons and members. This information can be obtained by calling your SNA, other nursing associations with legislative programs, your local League of Women Voters, or the local headquarters of your political party. Your state legislator's office will also be able to help you identify key people.

State judicial systems also influence how laws are implemented. On February 14, 1974, a district court judge in the District of Columbia ruled in the case of *Dixon v. Weinberger* that mentally handicapped people have "a statutory right to treatment in the least restrictive setting."[2] With this court decision as a standard, advocates of the mentally handicapped began to lobby state legislatures to establish policies that would further the deinstitutionalization of the retarded and mentally ill.

In Maryland the General Assembly's leadership appointed a joint committee (of which I was a member) to review state policies, programs, and services for the mentally handicapped. After 2 years of intensive work the committee recommended that the state fund community programs and services that would allow patients from mental hospitals and resident facilities for the retarded to be treated outside the walls of these institutions. Budgets did increase, but not fast enough to satisfy the well-organized lobbyists advocating deinstitutionalization, who appealed to the Maryland attorney general at that time, Steven Sachs. He became an advocate for the group of mentally retarded persons who had been inappropriately placed in mental institutions. He became such a strong advocate that these people were referred to as "the Sachs' population."

In Maryland it was ultimately the pressure from this high-ranking official and the judicial system that stimulated the state to move quickly through the budget and legislative process to establish the support systems required to treat mentally handicapped persons in the least restrictive setting.

THREE IMPORTANT STEPS IN THE DEVELOPMENT OF A LAW

To see how the legislative process works, let's follow the course a bill must take to become law. How does it move forward? What are the obstacles to getting it enacted? How and where can it "die" or be "killed"? What can proponents of a bill do to overcome these obstacles? Follow the illustration "How a bill becomes a law" on p. 88 as we review this important process. The illustration uses the bill-to-law process in Maryland as an example.

There are three important steps to enactment and implementation of a piece of legislation: passage by the legislature, signing by the governor, and establishment of rules and regulations for implementation. These steps vary little from state to state. Specific information about the bill-to-law procedures in your state can be obtained by calling or writing your state capitol (See Appendix C.), your local office of the League of Women Voters, or the local office of your political party. For a state-by-state comparison of these procedures, you can read Sarah E. Archer and Patricia A. Goehner's book, *Nurses: a political force.*[3] The nursing community's experience in attaining third-party payment for nurses in independent practice illustrates what may happen between conception of an idea and its enactment into law.

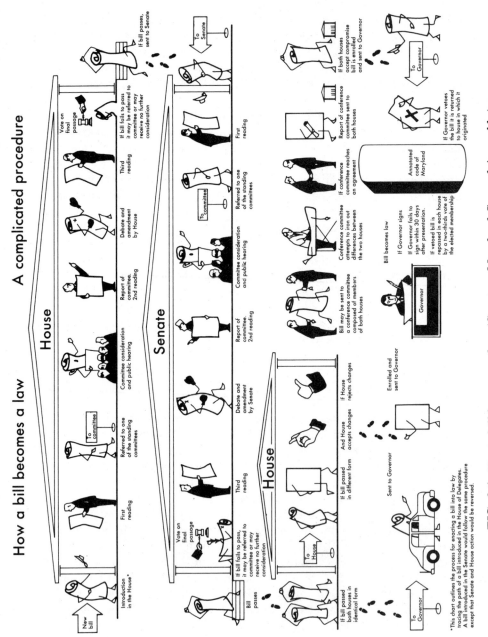

FIG. 6-1. How a bill becomes a law. (Courtesy Maryland General Assembly.)

ORIGINATION OF A BILL

People often wonder how ideas for laws are generated. Sometimes a legislator learns of a problem while speaking to a community group. But in most cases individuals or groups approach lawmakers with ideas for legislative solutions to problems. All that is required is a clear proposal backed up with appropriate data and information. From the legislator's viewpoint, the perception of each issue or cause boils down to the age-old question: What's in it for me? And by implication, what's in it for my constituents? Therefore as an advocate of a nursing or health care issue, you should be sure that a legislator sees immediately the many interests she or he has at stake.

In the case of our bill involving third-party payment, the idea came about in another way. I had read an article in the *American Journal of Nursing* about two nurses in New York State who opened a private practice but soon found they were unable to continue because insurance companies would not compensate them for their services. Clients whose health insurance contracts covered services that nurses were legally authorized to provide were denied coverage unless the services were provided by a physician.

I believed this practice denied the consumer the freedom to select the provider of his or her choice. It was unfair to both the consumer who wished to use the services of a nurse and the qualified nurse-provider. I wondered if there were legal barriers to the establishment of independent practices by qualified registered nurses in Maryland. My research showed that because Maryland's Nurse Practice Act specifically dictated the constraints of advanced practice, the only barrier was the economic one imposed by the insurance companies.

I believe it is important for all individuals to operate at their highest possible level. To set up restrictions that force any nurse to function at a level lower than that which is justified by her or his clinical training, skills, and education is an injustice to that person, a disservice to the public, and a roadblock to the professionalization of nursing. Those nurses willing and eager to assume the responsibilities of operating independently should be encouraged to do so. In a day when cost containment was becoming a watchword in the health care industry, the insurance companies' practice of denying compensation represented a wasteful failure to utilize valuable health care resources.

PREPARATION FOR DRAFTING OF A BILL

Members of the nursing community and I spent 6 months preparing for the drafting of the bill I introduced into the Maryland House of Delegates on February 10, 1977. We had three purposes in mind: to provide a method of tapping our valuable nursing resources, to provide consumers with a choice, and to provide economic assistance to those nurse-midwives and nurse-practitioners who want to practice independently.

The first bill would have required insurance companies to reimburse directly both nurse-midwives and nurse-practitioners for their services. Support came from a number of self-employed nurse-practitioners and nurse-midwives, the secretary of the Maryland Department of Health and Mental Hygiene (a physician), the Maryland Board of Examiners of Nurses (now called the Maryland Board of Nursing), the Visiting Nurse Association, and the Maryland Nurses' Association. In addition we were able to list a number of national groups, including the American Council of Life Insurance and Health Insurance Associations of America, who supported the principle of the bill.

It was not a great surprise that three dissenting voices were heard: Blue Shield of Maryland, the Board of Medical Examiners, and the Medical and Chirurgical Faculty of Maryland (the Maryland medical society).

As the chief sponsor of the bill, I looked for cosponsors—valuable assets in the effort to pass legislation—among my fellow delegates. At first, it was difficult to find them because the bill represented a very new idea. Few of my legislative colleagues at that time understood the role of the registered nurse in the modern health care delivery system. But in spite of the lack of understanding, I was eventually able to attract a few cosponsors. Because of their feeling of ownership of a bill, cosponsors will work for its passage by lobbying other legislators to vote for it.

In spite of the newness of the concept, nurses' testimony before the Committee on Economic Matters, the committee to which the bill had been assigned, was well received. We built a convincing case, but for a variety of reasons legislators were reluctant to pass the bill at that time and instead voted to study the issue over the summer.

It became obvious during the study of the first bill that legislators were unclear about what nurse-midwives and nurse-practitioners are prepared to do. We found that it was easier for them to understand the work of nurse-midwives, who have historically practiced independently. Since nurse-midwives' practices center around healthy processes—normal pregnancies, deliveries, and postpartum recoveries—it was easier to define it as separate from medicine. In fact, about that time, the California Court of Appeals ruled that the practice of midwifery is not in violation of the California medical licensing statute. The court made the point that pregnancy does not constitute an illness and that, therefore, the practice of midwifery is not the practice of medicine.

As a matter of strategy, I split the bill the next year, introducing one for nurse-midwives and a second for nurse-practitioners. I assumed it would be easier to pass the nurse-midwife bill and that once it became law, the stage would be set to attain reimbursement for nurse-practitioners. The strategy worked. We were able to pass the nurse-midwife bill in 1978 and the nurse-practitioner bill in 1979.

In 1984 the Association of Nurse Anesthetists asked me to introduce a reimbursement bill for them. The hearing on the bill was quite a contrast to those held on the earlier bills: Committee members were comfortable with the issues, and in fact the three opponents of the early bills testified in favor of

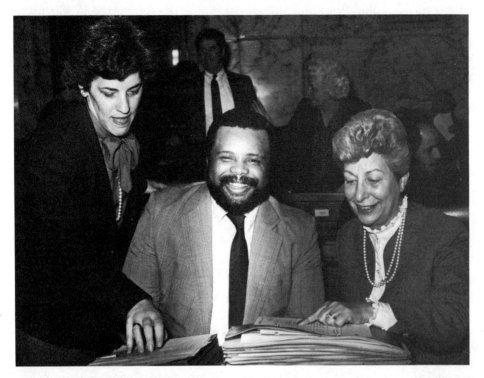

Delegate Nancy Kopp (left) and Delegate Marilyn Goldwater (right) discuss the nurse-midwife bill with Delegate Larry Young, Chairman of the Economic and Environmental Affairs Committee in January 1978.

passage of the latest bill. It sailed through both houses of the legislature without a dissenting vote.

INTRODUCTION OF A BILL

Regardless of the origin of the idea, when a legislator decides to introduce a bill, his or her first step is to request that the lawyers and issue specialists on the legislature's bill-drafting unit translate the idea into legal, technical, and constitutional language. The bill then serves as a vehicle for the legislators' discussion of the issue. On the basis of this discussion, legislative action may be deemed appropriate, or it may be found that the bill's objective can be achieved through budgetary or administrative action.

Once a bill is drafted, it is given a number, for example, House Bill 586 (HB

586) or Senate Bill 890 (SB 890). Bills are numbered consecutively in the order of their introduction. Presiding officers determine the committee to which the bill will be assigned, usually on the basis of its subject matter. The bill then receives its first reading in its sponsor's chamber, which is thereafter called the bill's "chamber of origin." The bill's title, number, and committee assignment are read, as are its main contents.

The committee hearing is perhaps a bill's first real test. The group of citizens who originally voiced a need for the proposed legislation usually provides people to testify. The bill's sponsor calls upon them, organizes testimony, and notifies people scheduled to testify of the day, time, and place of the hearing. (There are ways to prepare and deliver effective testimony, and we will talk about them in the next chapter.)

After hearing testimony, the committee schedules a work session, during which the testimony, proposed amendments, and other relevant information are discussed. On the basis of suggestions from witnesses or through ideas developed during the work session, committee members may propose amendments at this time.

Amendments, which can be made at any time during a bill's progress to enactment, may enhance or may gut a bill. An example of a crippling amendment is one proposed during the work session of our third-party–payment bill by a legislator with backing from insurance and medical lobbies. His amendment would have required that for a nurse to be compensated by an insurance company, a physician would have to refer the client and supervise the nurse. Such a change would have eliminated the reason for the bill: to allow nurses autonomy in practice. I led the argument against the proposed amendment, and fortunately enough committee members had the good sense to vote it down.

Once study of a bill is complete, the committee votes on the bill and reports it out. The vote may be "favorable," "favorable with amendments," or "unfavorable." If the committee votes "unfavorable," no discussion takes place on the chamber's floor and the bill dies. If the bill receives a "favorable" or "favorable with amendments" vote, the chairperson of the committee reports the vote to the floor, and debate on the bill usually follows. During this debate, members of the chamber can offer amendments. The process of reporting it out and discussing it on the chamber floor is called the second reading. Ultimately a second-reading vote is taken. If the bill passes, it is then printed in its final form with all adopted amendments incorporated. (See examples in the Appendix.)

Once printed with all the changes, the bill comes back for a third reading and final vote. Debate may occur again, but no amendments may be made. At this point legislators must give the bill a straight "yes" or "no" vote. If it is defeated, the bill dies, at least for that legislative session. If it passes, the bill is sent to the second chamber, where it goes through the same process. In this chamber, however, the bill may be amended on third reading (a significant difference from the procedure in the first chamber).

If amendments are added in the second chamber, the bill is sent back to the committee to which it was originally assigned in the first chamber. This committee can accept or reject amendments added by the other chamber. The committee chairperson explains the committee's position on the floor of the chamber, and once more the issues are debated. If the amendments are rejected in the first chamber, the bill goes to a conference committee, made up of members of both chambers appointed by each chamber's presiding officer.

The conference committee meets to work out differences if they can. Members report back to their respective chambers. Their action must then be approved by a majority vote of the members of both houses. When members of the conference committee agree, the bill usually is ratified by both houses. If they disagree, the bill dies.

Once a bill is passed by both houses, it goes to the governor to be signed. If he or she chooses to sign it, the bill becomes law. But even after the bill goes to the governor to be signed, it may be in jeopardy of failing. Opponents of the bill may ask for a veto hearing. The governor, having studied the issues, may decide to veto the bill with or without a hearing. When vetoing a piece of legislation, he or she must give reasons for the decision. The legislature may vote to disagree with, or override, the governor's veto. In most states an override requires the vote of more than a straight majority of the members of both houses; usually a two-thirds or three-fifths majority is required.

Assuming the governor plans to sign the bill, he or she, the legislative sponsors, and the bill's proponents often use the bill-signing ceremony to make a positive public statement. Such ceremonies are momentous occasions for all of the people who worked for the passage of the legislation. In Maryland the governor, the president of the Senate, the speaker of the House, and the secretary of state all must sign the bill. During the ceremony, they are seated at a table with backers of the bill behind them. Representatives of both the print and electronic media are also present. Once the bill is signed, the governor presents the signing pen to the chief sponsor of the legislation. It is difficult to describe the sense of triumph that Maryland nurses, other proponents of the bill, and I felt when the bills involving third-party payment for nurses in independent practice were signed and we realized that our efforts had been successful. (See photograph of bill-signing ceremony on p. 137.)

To reach this point, however, proponents of a bill have to be persistent and creative. As you can see, opponents of a piece of legislation have ample opportunity to block its passage. At one point during the progress of our bill involving third-party payment, the bill was temporarily stuck in conference committee. The committee's chairman opposed the bill and was prepared to let it die there in the closing hours of the legislative session. He suddenly disappeared. I realized that he was making himself unavailable to me by staying in the men's room. I pushed the Speaker to insist he come out and hold the meeting. Under pressure, the chairman came out. The committee worked out a compromise, and the bill received a "favorable" vote at 11:55 PM the last night of the session. The MNA lobbyist at that time, Lynelle King, and I were too tired to celebrate.

IMPLEMENTATION OF THE LAW

Once a bill becomes law, its proponents must still take steps to ensure that it is implemented as intended. The agency under whose jurisdiction the law will fall can make a crucial difference as to whether the law's implementation reflects the intention of its backers.

The power of government agencies is reflected in the comments of Carolyne K. Davis, who administered the HCFA from 1981 to 1985. Federal agencies such as the HCFA have a great influence on health policy. To illustrate the point, Davis says:

> The agency develops a legislative agenda, as well as the budget that will support the agency's activities. Long-range planning occurs through research and demonstration. Successful demonstrations are apt to be adopted as a new health policy later. HCFA is also responsible for implementation of rules and regulations implementing health care legislation. The administration [HCFA] makes decisions in each of these areas. And in addition the agency can control the time table (to some extent) as to when implementation will occur.[4]

State boards of nursing carry out their business on the basis of nurse practice acts and other legislation affecting the profession. They develop the regulations that put the laws into practice. For instance, their regulations dictate how schools of nursing are certified, how nurses are registered, how nursing practice is defined, what nursing functions can and cannot be delegated, and how disciplinary hearings are held.

At both the federal and state levels, the agency that will administer the law develops the regulations to implement it. And these regulations have the force of law, so they should reflect the spirit, as well as the language, of the enacted law. Therefore, as regulations are being developed, the proponents of a law must be observant. In most states, regulations must be published for the information of the public before they are adopted. Public hearings are held. There is a period in which any individual is free to comment and to influence the adoption or content of regulations. Call or write your state capitol for information about how regulations are published in your state. If you are interested in a specific bill, ask for the time and place of public hearings.

Implementation of a law may require the cooperation of more than one agency, so there are procedures that prevent regulations made by one agency from conflicting with those made by another. In the case of our bill to attain third-party payment, both the Board of Nursing and the Department of Licensing and Regulation (which regulates the insurance industry) were involved in the development of the regulations required by this new legislation.

Once the law had passed and the regulations were promulgated, insurance companies sent out forms making it possible for nurses to sign up for provider numbers, which are required for reimbursement. It was called to my attention that Blue Shield of Maryland had sent out forms including a space for the signature of "the supervising physician." I believed that this requirement violated the intent of the law, so I argued that the legislation did not require a supervising physician and, therefore, that the insurance company had no authority to ask for a physician's signature. I brought the issue to the attention of the insurance commissioner, who in turn asked the attorney general to review the form and the law. The attorney general agreed with me. The commissioner then told Blue Shield to recall the forms and send out new ones, deleting the offending phrase.

The procedures required to establish the regulations that implement laws are laborious and time-consuming. Donna Dorsey, the executive director of the Maryland Board of Nursing, said, "In Maryland the whole process takes approximately 6 months—if all goes smoothly."

A great deal happens between the time of a bill's conception and its implementation. The success we and others have had in gaining insurance payment for independent nurses' services shows what nurses can do when we work together. As the largest group of health care providers, nurses have tremendous potential strength in the political and legislative arenas—strength that until recently has been largely unrealized.

As the conference committee voted for passage of the bill mandating third-party payment to nurse-midwives, the lobbyist for Blue Shield was heard saying to the medical society's lobbyist: "Goldwater has awakened the sleeping giant— the nursing profession is on the move."

By July 1988, 28 states had at least some sort of legislation under their state health insurance laws that mandated third-party payment for some categories of nurses in advanced practice.[5] This type of legislation and any other that will benefit the nursing profession and the public's access to health care are attainable in any state if certain elements are in place: First, nurses must be knowledgeable about the legislative process and how it works. They must have their goals clearly conceptualized and be prepared to communicate them forcefully. They must have the facts and figures to back up their positions and to turn aside their opponents' arguments. Nursing leadership must be committed to making something happen. There must be grass-roots commitment and organization that includes both nursing and consumer groups interested in health care. Finally, sponsors and all supporters of the legislation must demonstrate determination, tenacity, and perseverance.

REFERENCES

1. Annual Insurance Report—1986-1987, Washington, D.C., 1988, U.S. Office of Personnel Management.
2. *Dixon v Weinberger,* 74285 (District of Columbia district court 1974).
3. Archer SE and Goehner PA: Nurses: a political force, Monterey, Calif, 1982, Wadsworth, Inc, Health Sciences Division.
4. Davis CK: Personal communication, December 1987.
5. McCloughlin S (ANA): Personal communication, July 1988.

Chapter 7

⫻ LOBBYING FOR POLITICAL INFLUENCE

Lobbying is part of the art of influencing people. A lobbyist's job at any level of government is to influence the outcome of proposed legislation in favor of the clients and causes the lobbyist represents.

In spite of its image of power, there should be nothing mystifying or frightening about lobbying. Some people assume that lobbying is somehow dishonest and that to be effective, lobbyists must have large amounts of money available to wine and dine legislators. Actually, the merits of a cause and the amount of backing constituents can gain in the legislature are more important than money. Because of the urgency of their causes, representatives of vulnerable groups, such as the homeless, the retarded, and the mentally ill, are frequently very effective—even when their organizations' budgets are limited. Their strength is pulling on legislators' heartstrings and gathering the votes of their causes' supporters at election time. Lobbying is an honorable activity, and anyone can do it. Sally Austen Tom, a former lobbyist for the American College of Nurse-Midwives, has said, "Lobbyists are the only people in Washington who are honest about what they do."[1]

In contrast to the U.S. Congress, which is essentially in session all year, most state legislatures meet for a limited time annually. In Maryland the session lasts just 90 days, from mid-January to mid-April. In that short time, 3,000 to 4,000 bills are introduced. Of these, approximately 10% are health related. (States' budgets are also involved with health issues, since they provide funding for state health services.) In their attempt to deal with all of these matters, legislators must face frantic sessions of work, study, and action. In this pressured setting, lobbying is vital.

Good lobbyists earn legislators' respect because they supply accurate information. A legislator wants facts to support his or her position on an issue and to know the points the opposition will make and the best way to counter them. A good lobbyist is able to present the arguments on both sides of an issue. You can be sure that a lobbyist who supplies false information to a legislator will never be welcome again in that legislator's office.

Lobbying can be done at many different levels. Professional lobbyists represent such disparate interests as nurses, teachers, physicians, labor unions, and the tobacco and oil industries. Citizen lobbyists represent groups who organize around issues or segments of the population with special needs, such as the environment or the interests of elderly persons. Constituents frequently lobby on particular issues during the time these issues are being debated. In a sense, anyone who attempts to influence a legislator could be called a lobbyist. If you have ever written a letter to or talked with a legislator about an issue or responded to a request from an interest group to join its campaign by mailing a card to a particular legislator, you have lobbied.

Some lobbyists are highly paid, some modestly so, and many not at all. The media often focus on the highly paid representatives of industry and business. But lower-paid lobbyists, volunteers, or people who bring individual concerns directly to their legislators make up the majority of lobbyists, especially in state legislatures. A legislator's constituents have special clout: while business and industry can bring a legislator needed campaign money, constituents can bring votes—an equally important ingredient in winning an election.

LOBBYING OUTSIDE AND INSIDE THE LEGISLATURE

"External lobbying" refers to all activities occurring outside the legislature that increase the visibility of an issue in the public arena. It includes all grass-roots efforts aimed at influencing governmental decisions, as well as efforts to influence public opinion and build consensus, such as letters to the editor, press conferences, and activities that attract the media. During the 1980s organized groups of citizens have grown and "matured." They have become more articulate in presenting their causes and more sophisticated in building support for their positions. Groups such as the Sierra Club (which lobbies for environmental causes), the American Association of Retired Persons, and NOW are examples of such organizations employing more sophisticated tactics.

External Lobbying: One Successful Effort

An excellent example of external lobbying on a local level is the efforts of a coalition of women's groups in Montgomery County, Maryland. In 1980 under the leadership of the Montgomery County Commission on Women, the legislative committees of the local chapters of several women's organizations banded together to gain more power and influence on issues of mutual interest. The groups included chapters of the League of Women Voters, NOW, and the Maryland Nurses' Association.

Determined to mold public opinion on women's issues and to promote legislation that would benefit women and their families, the groups planned a "Women's Legislative Briefing," to which they invited legislators, the press, and all interested citizens. (Men were included, since the position was taken that "women's issues" are really "people's issues," meaning that everything that affects women affects everyone else in society.) This first briefing was so successful that it was held again the following year. The briefings have since become annual events with increasing support. The county executive or another prominent local official is invited to speak at the briefings. The events address issues such as child care, comparable worth, and the effect of tax policy on working mothers.

What was started by a small group of organizers representing 12 different women's organizations in our area has expanded to include groups not only from our own county but also from our neighbor, Prince George's County. More than 60 organizations sponsored the 1988 briefing. These highly visible forums influence both legislators and the public on issues of particular interest to women.

Lobbying within the Legislature

Internal lobbying, or lobbying within the legislature, is more direct. It consists of personal contact between legislators and lobbyists or constituents through telephone calls, letters, or visits to legislators' offices.

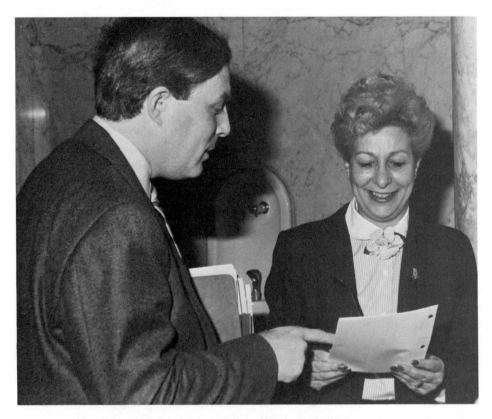

A lobbyist catches Delegate Goldwater in the halls of the state capitol.

In Maryland, opportunities for citizens to lobby lawmakers directly during the legislative session are expanded through weekly Citizens' Nights at the Legislature. In contrast to other days of the week, the Legislature conducts its sessions in the evening on Mondays, allowing more citizens with daytime commitments to see their representatives in action. These evenings are always exciting. Highly paid professional lobbyists rub shoulders with citizen lobbyists who have come to promote their causes. The galleries, halls, and balconies are filled with people seeking opportunities to talk with their legislators, to influence them, or merely to observe them at work. It is a little like Parent Teacher Association–sponsored back-to-school nights, but instead of opportunities for parents to talk with teachers, citizens have opportunities to talk with their elected representatives.

A more substantial form of internal lobbying is to testify before a committee, and we will talk more about how to do this effectively later in this chapter.

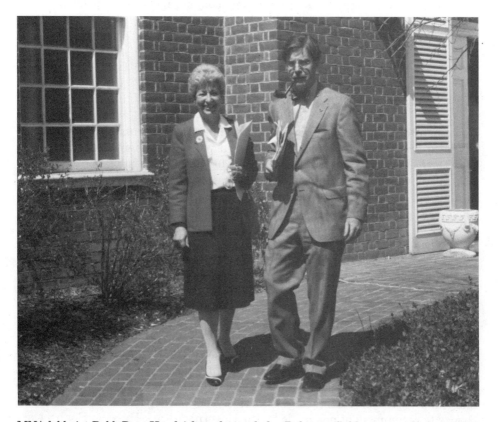

MNA lobbyist Robb Ross Hendrickson buttonholes Delegate Goldwater as she leaves the House Office Building.

Since most work in any legislature is done while bills are before committee, that is the time when lobbying efforts are most effective. Committee decisions carry a lot of weight when a bill goes to the floor. Only when a controversial bill comes out of committee with a close vote is there an opportunity to influence the rest of the chamber on an issue. Although it does happen occasionally, a committee decision is rarely overturned.

Lobbyists become skilled at counting those legislators who support them on a bill, those who don't, and those who are undecided. During the times when a vote is imminent, lobbyists' most intense efforts are directed toward legislators whose votes are undecided.

The ANA and most national nursing organizations have paid lobbyists in Washington. Most SNAs and many specialty nursing organizations now have them at their state capitols, at least while the legislature is in session. The presence of these lobbyists in the halls of Congress and state legislatures represents nursing's interest in sharing power with other health care providers in the making of public health care policy. It is one sign of nursing's political coming of age. Later in this chapter we will discuss lobbying methods that nurses have found to be effective in influencing legislative outcomes. But before we do, let's look at how government officials—both executives and legislators—lobby each other.

HOW GOVERNMENT OFFICIALS LOBBY EACH OTHER

Enactment of a legislative program is a complex process, and citizen and paid lobbyists are not the only ones engaged in promoting their causes. In every capital, the governor and his staff attempt to persuade members of the legislature to enact programs they've developed, the leadership of each party attempts to influence its members to vote for the legislation it endorses, and legislators constantly lobby each other.

How the Executive Lobbies

Neither a President of the United States nor a state governor, as chief executive, can initiate legislation. But presidents and governors have powerful influence that goes far beyond the simple authority to sign or veto a bill. Using his leadership position, a president or a governor can actively campaign for legislation he supports. In some cases, he may propose legislation, and his staff of experts may actually draft it. Once drafted, he then asks the leaders of Congress or, in the case of a governor, the state legislature, to introduce the legislation.

A president or governor can lobby the legislature in many ways. In 1985 Maryland Governor Harry Hughes actively backed legislation drafted in response to recommendations made by the Governor's Task Force on Health Care Cost Containment. His staff participated in legislative committee work sessions in an effort to refine language to satisfy legislators. After many hours of work the legislators, with the help of the governor's staff, were able to draft bills that controlled costs and still provided Maryland citizens access to high-quality health care. The bills were so well constructed in committee that there was little debate on the floor. In both houses the bills passed unchanged.

In other instances the governor may lobby individual legislators directly. It is not uncommon for a legislator to receive a call from the governor's office saying, "The governor wanted me to talk to you about the . . . bill." At this point the governor's representative will point out the benefits of the proposed legislation to the people living in the legislator's district and tell the lawmaker that the governor hopes he or she will vote for the bill. If the governor knows the vote will be close, he may actually call undecided legislators into his office to try to convince them to adopt his point of view and vote his way.

Such was the case when a bill raising the drinking age from 18 to 21 years was introduced into the Maryland legislature in 1982. Supporters believed the bill would help decrease the number of drunken-driving accidents. Opponents believed that citizens old enough to be drafted for military service were old enough to use their own judgment regarding their ability to drink and drive. Governor Hughes knew the bill was controversial and the vote was likely to be close because many legislators were undecided. He started calling groups of them into his office to persuade them to support the bill. In this case the governor had substantial support from citizen groups outside the legislature. Mothers Against Drunk Driving, Students Against Driving Drunk, critical care nurses, emergency medicine physicians, and many other interested citizens worked for passage of the bill.

Before the bill was brought up for a vote, the leaders (whips) of both the House and Senate took counts. As soon as they knew that enough legislators intended to support the bill, they called for a vote. The bill passed.

How Party Leadership Lobbies

At the beginning of every legislative session the leadership of each party meets to determine its legislative priorities. The elected and appointed officers of both chambers and committee chairpersons (or important members of committees in the case of the minority party) meet to set each party's agenda for the session.

Both parties closely examine the program outlined by the chief executive. At the federal level the president presents his program in the State of the Union address, which he delivers before both houses of Congress, distinguished guests, and millions of people watching on television. In most state governments the governor sets forth his program at the opening of a legislative session in a similar address before the state's lawmakers. In almost all cases the chief executive's party will support his program, while the opposing party will examine it more critically, often proposing alternative programs.

Party whips are given their assignments at the beginning of each session. Each is given a certain number of legislators with whom to keep in contact as issues come up. Whips must constantly be aware of how individuals in their assigned groups feel about positions the party leadership takes on various issues. The whips take concerns back to the floor leaders and work for the accommodation of differences when they arise.

During the last 2 years of my tenure in the Maryland House of Delegates, I served as deputy majority whip. What happened in 1983 illustrates the challenges and excitement involved with this position. A bill seeking to curb the soaring costs of state government by limiting automatic cost-of-living increases for state employees was introduced. The majority party's leaders and others who supported the bill believed that continued automatic cost-of-living increases could bankrupt the state. However, many legislators opposed the proposal because they felt the measure would hurt retirees. The bill became very controversial as it was debated on the floor.

Whips were sent out to count votes, to make sure that those supporting the bill had not changed their minds, and to check with the undecided legislators. When talking with undecided legislators, I would simply ask if they had made a decision yet, if they needed any information to help them decide, and if they had concerns or suggestions they wanted me to share at leadership meetings. I asked if they wanted me to check back with them or if they would let me know when they had made a final decision. I would end the conversation by saying, "The leadership really needs your support on this bill."

The bill was finally called up for a vote, and tension was high as the votes were counted. The bill passed by one vote—a close call.

Being a party whip is a leadership position that involves pressure—but also excitement and satisfaction when you win.

The Caucuses

Within every legislature, several groups with similar interests organize caucuses to reach certain goals. The Democratic and Republican parties form caucuses in each chamber of Congress and each state legislature. Members choose party leaders and attempt to persuade each other to vote with the party on crucial issues.

In recent years caucuses have been organized to benefit special populations. For example, in addition to the bipartisan Women's Caucus in Congress, 11 state legislatures had women's caucuses in 1988.* The number of states with such caucuses varies slightly from year to year. Many states do not have enough women in the legislature to form them, and in some states such caucuses are looked upon as divisive. Women in other states elected not to form them for other political reasons. Women's caucuses have lobbied for the reform of rape laws, equitable distribution of marital property, equal pay for equal work, programs to decrease infant mortality, improvements in child care services and prenatal care, and tax policies to help working mothers.

---

*These states included Alaska, California, Connecticut, Illinois, Iowa, Kansas, Maryland, Massachusetts, New York, North Carolina, and Virginia.[2]

Similarly, black caucuses have been organized in Congress and in several state legislatures. They have benefited their constituents by lobbying for assistance to businesses run by minorities, expansion of minority employment, and cost-effective, quality health care programs and services for minorities.

The goals of different groups may be in conflict at some times but may blend with those of other groups at other times. When groups are in agreement, they often form loose coalitions and work for a common goal.

Legislators Lobby Each Other

In addition to the proposals for legislation developed by the executive branch, party leaders, and special-interest caucuses, legislators themselves have ideas for bills, many of which are drafted and then introduced in either house of the legislature.

Legislators are constantly trying to influence each other in an attempt to build support for legislation they have sponsored or for bills backed by their party. Some legislators develop expertise on certain issues, and their colleagues call on them for advice on these issues, because they are known to be knowledgeable. This was the case with me when health care issues arose.

In some cases votes are traded. This practice is not as corrupt as might be imagined. When I wanted votes for my bill to gain insurance payment to nurses in advanced practice, I worked with my colleagues from the rural sections of Maryland—the areas near the Chesapeake Bay and in mountainous western Maryland. The concerns of many of their constituents—farmers, watermen, lumbermen—were different from the concerns of my constituents in suburban Washington, D.C. If their proposed legislation did not compromise my principles and would not hurt my constituents, I was willing to vote for their bills—if they would vote for mine. These agreements helped me gather enough votes for passage of my bills.

WHERE DO NURSES FIT IN?

Where, then, do nurses find a place in this crazy quilt of lobbying? How can nurses establish positions on issues? How can they organize? And how can they gain attention and develop support for their issues?

The most effective lobbying involves group effort. Most nursing organizations have legislative committees, formed by a committed group of nurses interested in promoting nursing and health-policy goals through legislation. They meet regularly, especially during the time the legislature is in session, to study bills affecting these health care areas. Relevant bills are assigned to the members of the committee. At least one person studies each bill thoroughly, trying to get all the facts about the bill, as well as all the arguments for and against it. This person presents her findings to the members of the group, who then debate the issues before taking a stand. Association lobbyists participate in the discussions and provide political advice. Many nurses' associations not only take a position for or against a bill but also rate it as to how heavily the organization will lobby on it. High priority ratings guide rank-and-file association members to the bills for which the organization wants the greatest efforts expended. Since events move quickly, there is obviously a limited amount of time for making these decisions.

The first step in understanding and taking action on a bill is reading it. Reading a bill for the first time is like tackling a foreign language, because bills are drafted in language that complies with legal and constitutional standards. The "Explanation to facilitate reading of legislative bills," found in Appendix D, will help you understand this style. Use it to read the examples of a Third Reader House Joint Resolution, a First Reader Senate Bill, and a Third Reader Senate Bill, found on pp. 190-194. Then read the final version of the Maryland bill on pp. 195-201 to mandate insurance payment to nurse-midwives. This is the form in which the bill was sent to the governor for his signature. You will find that at each stage a bill looks a little different, but reading one is not so difficult after all.

Examples and explanations of other documents, found in Appendix D, will help you understand how legislators and their staffs receive information about the status of bills and schedules of upcoming events. These documents include the Daily Synopsis of Bills and Resolutions Introduced in the (Maryland) House of Delegates, a committee report, and a Third Reading Calendar.

After reading it, what should a person studying a bill consider when deciding whether to support or oppose it? You will want to ask yourself and the members of your nursing organization's legislative committee these questions (as well as others): What problem does the bill address? What effect will discussion of the problem have on the problem? If enacted, how will legislation solve the problem? How will the new law be implemented? Who will be affected by it? And if it will cost money, how will a new program be financed? Help is available for resolving financial questions. When a bill is introduced, the fiscal department of the legislature analyzes the cost of implementing the proposed changes by looking at both the anticipated expenditures and revenues. This information is available to the public in the form of a Fiscal Note (See example in Appendix D.) and will be important to you in making an intelligent decision whether to support or oppose a bill.

Once you and your committee take a stand, the results of all of your study will have a second use: you and your colleagues will use the facts and figures again when you begin to lobby.

ORGANIZING TESTIMONY

If you or your group plans to lobby intensely on a bill, you will want to present testimony at the legislative committee's hearing. And you will want to organize this testimony for maximum effect. If several people are to testify, the group's effort must be coordinated. Each person can present one argument in support of the group's position, or one person can present all the arguments. But before beginning testimony, that person should ask the rest of the group to stand so that it is clear to the legislators that the person presenting testimony speaks for a substantial number of people. Members of the group may be introduced to show the commitment and diversity of members of the nursing community who support the group's position. This introduction should include names and professional credentials.

When I introduced my third-party–payment bill in the Maryland House of Delegates, my nursing colleagues and I wanted to make an impression on the other legislators. We wanted nurses to provide a show of support by being there in large numbers. We asked them to wear white uniforms with stethoscopes around their necks. Ordinarily, nurses would not wear their uniforms while lobbying, but in this case we believed that a large number of highly visible nurses would capture the legislators' attention. Our strategy worked; the show of white piqued the lawmakers' interest.

We planned a forceful presentation, realizing that this was our best opportunity to lobby the legislative committee as a whole. I opened the testimony with a brief statement about the purpose of the bill. Then each nurse-midwife and nurse-practitioner gave one reason why the bill would benefit consumers, the health care delivery system, and the nursing profession. Each nurse's testimony was substantive. Each one emphasized the possible financial savings coming from broadened use of nurses in the health care delivery system. Each nurse made the point that nurses can provide cost-effective, quality health care. After completing her testimony, each nurse provided committee members with a typewritten copy of it and included copies of appropriate background material to support our point of view.

After the hearing, nurses visited both committee members and legislators from their districts, promoting the bill and providing informational packets to those who had not received them during the hearing. They lobbied so aggres-

---

Keys to Presenting Effective Testimony to a Legislative Committee

- Have the facts well organized.
- Be familiar with your testimony so you will not have to read it.
- Be brief. State your point in the first paragraph, expand on it in the second paragraph, and summarize it in the third paragraph.
- Speak in terms your audience will understand. Most legislators are not nurses. Do not use nursing jargon, which is unintelligible to most lay people.
- Have enough typewritten copies of your testimony and supportive background material available to give to all members of the committee.

sively and were so visible in the halls of the Capitol that one of my fellow legislators said, "I never thought I'd want to hide from a nurse." When the bill went to the other chamber, nurses made the same effort there. Throughout the process, they wrote letters and telephoned not only their own legislators but also key members of the committees studying the bill. The lobbying campaign was very effective. Legislators were impressed by the merits of their arguments and the commitment and professionalism of the nurses. The bill passed.

To be successful, testimony must be presented forcefully and articulately, and the information given must be accurate. (Keys to presenting effective testimony are given in the box on p. 105.)

DIRECT LOBBYING

The time for the most intensive lobbying is after the committee hearing and before the work and study session. Keep in mind the suggestions for giving effective testimony when you visit a legislator's office; they are important during this next step in the lobbying process. Be well organized, knowledgeable, clear, and, by all means, brief. Present one or, at the most, two ideas. Come back with a third later, and only if it is necessary. Remember that people constantly approach legislators with ideas, so your idea must be presented concisely to be remembered. Provide written material that explains your idea more fully. Be sure to include facts and figures in usable form. You may write to or call committee members about a bill before or after the hearing, as long as you do it before the committee votes.

When a bill comes out of committee, try to determine how it will do in the chamber by asking members of the committee or the nursing association's lobbyist. Any one of these people should be able to tell you whether lobbying is necessary. If it is deemed important, urge nurses to contact the legislators from their districts. Telephone trees are the most effective way to mobilize rank-and-file lobbying efforts quickly. One person calls a specified number of people, asking them to carry out a certain action—in this case, letting their legislators know their position on a bill. Let's say this person makes five calls. Each of the people she reaches will then call five others. This process continues until a substantial number of people have been called.

When writing or telephoning your legislator regarding a bill, state your position concisely. A letter written by you in your own words will be more effective than any form letter, but there are styles to follow for addressing letters to government officials. (See the accompanying box for the appropriate forms.)

Telephone and mail campaigns lend support to witnesses and their information, but they cannot be used in place of other lobbying. They back up personal lobbying but are not by themselves effective ways to influence a legislator. What such campaigns do is alert legislators that an issue is important to a group of constituents.

Form letters that require only a signature (the type sent out by many

Styles for Addressing Correspondence to Government Officials

Styles for the inside address and envelope are given first; the salutation follows.

U.S. SENATOR
The Honorable _____
United States Senate
Senate Office Building
Washington, D.C. 20510

Dear Senator _____

REPRESENTATIVE IN THE U.S. HOUSE OF REPRESENTATIVES
The Honorable _____
The United States House of Representatives
House Post Office
Washington, D.C. 20515

Dear Mr., Mrs., Ms. _____

GOVERNOR
The Honorable _____
Governor, State of _____
Capitol Building
City, State, Zip Code

Dear Governor _____

STATE SENATOR
The Honorable _____
Senator, _____ District
Capitol Building
City, State, Zip Code

Dear Senator _____

STATE REPRESENTATIVE
The Honorable _____
Representative (or Delegate or Member of the Assembly),
_____ District
State House of Representatives (or State House of Delegates or State Assembly)
Capitol Building
City, State, Zip Code

Dear Mr., Mrs., Ms. _____

special-interest groups) fall into this category. At one time an animal-rights group mounted an ambitious campaign in the Maryland legislature to outlaw the use of animals in medical research. Within a week my office took 425 telephone calls, some of them from as far away as California. I received 700 pieces of mail—most of them form postcards. I recognized the effort for what it was: a well-organized campaign by a committed national organization focusing on a specific and rather narrow issue. While I appreciated the concerns expressed, I thought that people who do not live in the state in which the campaign is mounted may get better results from concentrating their energies on Congress or their own state legislatures, where they can be more effective.

CHOOSING PEOPLE TO LOBBY

When building support in the legislature for your position, remember that the committee chairperson is a key to success. He or she has a responsibility to all citizens, so winning the chairperson's support is vital. You will also want to lobby committee members and the legislators from your district. Remember that as a constituent you are especially important to your legislator. Contacts with the President of the Senate and the Speaker of the House are also useful. If they support your bill, they may use their influence to move it along.

When nursing organizations promote a legislative initiative, they should try to get sponsors in both houses. In general, nursing and health care are not partisan issues; therefore, cosponsors for bills should be obtained from among both the Democrats and Republicans. The ability to draw support from both political parties should work to nursing's advantage.

Nurses have a professional responsibility and an obligation to educate legislators. We cannot expect them to understand our concerns and needs or those of our clients unless we tell them. The reservoir of goodwill that nurses have developed with legislators through the activities described in Chapter 4 will help when you lobby on a special issue. These activities include developing contacts during nurse-sponsored receptions for legislators, holding meetings and workshops at which legislators are asked to speak, and sponsoring nurses' days at the state capitol. And everyday involvement in the community is always important for building rapport with legislators—a valuable asset when special issues arise.

Keep in mind that legislators are human. They respond to courtesy and personal recognition. Let them know when you appreciate what they have done by sending a thank-you note. (Such notes also help legislators to remember your name.)

NURSES AS PROFESSIONAL LOBBYISTS

Professional nurse-lobbyists have increased visibility on Capitol Hill and in state legislatures in recent years. One reason for the increased visibility is the

ANA, which opened its Washington, D.C., office in 1954 with one lobbyist. It now has a staff of 17, seven of whom are lobbyists. This expansion of the ANA's Washington office indicates the importance the organization now places on having representation in the halls of Congress and at federal agencies.

Although the ANA is the largest governmental affairs office in nursing, other national nursing organizations also have professional lobbyists in the nation's capital.* On a contract basis the ANA represents a number of other nursing organizations, including the American Association of Critical-Care Nurses, Association of Operating Room Nurses, International Association for Enterostomal Therapy, and the Association for Practitioners in Infection Control. These groups work effectively on many nursing issues in both formal and informal coalitions.

Donna Richardson, RN, JD, ANA Director of Congressional and Agency Relations, brought to her position several years' experience as an attorney for the Department of Labor's Solicitors Office, Division of Occupational Safety and Health Administration. In that position Richardson dealt with many of the issues important to nursing, including access to quality health care, equal employment and other labor issues, and occupational health, from another angle. Richardson says:

> At the agency people came to educate us regarding occupational health concerns. Now as a nurse-lobbyist I attempt to educate the policy-makers on general health and nursing issues.
>
> The ANA encourages nurses to become politically active, especially at the state and local level. We would like to see more nurses on public boards and commissions and holding elective and appointive offices. To encourage and educate nurses in the political-legislative arena, the ANA has informal internship programs for individual nurses and in connection with a number of university undergraduate and graduate nursing programs. We provide a training ground for nurses in health care lobbying at the federal and state levels, and we are pleased that some have gone on to work as health care analysts on congressional and agency staffs.[3]

In addition to the nurse-lobbyists working at the federal level, a significant number of SNAs and other nursing organizations employ nurse-lobbyists to represent them in state legislatures. And a few nurses now lobby for businesses with health care interests.

One such person is Deborah Smith-Callahan, RN, who began her career as a lobbyist for the Illinois Nurses' Association (INA) at the state capitol in Springfield. After a brief assignment in the Washington office of the ANA, she became the first woman to be hired by the state government relations department of Pfizer Pharmaceuticals. She now represents the company in five state legislatures, in Indiana, Kentucky, Michigan, Ohio, and West Virginia. She lobbies for full access to medication therapy for Medicaid recipients and focuses on the cost-effectiveness of appropriate care. One of the reasons Smith-Callahan accepted

---

*These organizations include the American Association of Nurse Anesthetists, Emergency Nurses Association, Nurses Association of the American College of Obstetricians and Gynecologists, American Association of Colleges of Nursing, American College of Nurse-Midwives, and the National Association of Pediatric Nurses Associates and Practitioners.

her present position was her desire to return to lobbying in state legislatures:

> State legislators and their staffs are very accessible, and an effective lobbyist can have a significant impact on the development of state policy. It's extremely gratifying to successfully promote legislation or regulations which ultimately result in better health care for that state's citizens.
>
> Nurses tend to possess excellent lobbying skills. We have a good image with legislators and their staffs. We are good communicators and have credibility on key health care issues.

She adds, however, that nursing organizations should not eliminate the possibility of hiring someone other than a nurse to lobby for them. "A good lobbyist must have the professional skills and the expertise to develop and implement critical legislative strategies. By the same token they must know when to call in nurses for expert advice and testimony."

She believes that all nurses should lobby for professional-practice issues and quality health care:

> Grass-roots lobbying and networking among nurses can greatly enhance our influence in state legislatures. We can maximize the influence of professional nursing by utilizing the resources we do have. These include the ability to present credible information and—in terms of political action—to provide reliable campaign volunteers for candidates who support professional nursing.[4]

Patricia Barnett, RN, JD, lobbies for ER Squibb & Sons, another pharmaceutical company, in nine state legislatures, including those in Illinois, Michigan, and Ohio. With so much territory to cover, she must concentrate on key states, especially those that may be trend-setters. Her issues are access to health care for Medicaid recipients, product liability, medical malpractice, and the implications of cutbacks in federal funding.

Barnett became involved in lobbying through her experience as director of the INA's Economic & General Welfare program. She and Smith-Callahan worked together in Springfield, Illinois. Barnett developed political-action units within her bargaining units and tried to educate nurses on not only how to negotiate a contract but also how collective bargaining is related to the legislative and political processes.[5]

Barbara Curtis, one of the founders of the ANA/PAC, has been a mentor for both Smith-Callahan and Barnett. Smith-Callahan says:

> Barb has used her practical political skills to bring about legislation that implements nursing ideals and initiatives, issues important to patients. By watching her, I have learned how to compromise without giving away those goals that are truly important. Barb has convinced me that professional nursing will eventually be one of the strongest voices at both the federal level and in every state legislature in the nation.[4]

MOBILIZING FOR SUCCESS

Nurses are now tapping previously unrealized sources of power within themselves and their profession. There is power in ideas and knowledge. There is power in experience and expertise. There is power in numbers and organization. We are knowledgeable on health care issues. We understand what goes on in practice settings. We understand what patients and their families need. We are their natural advocates.

The question is: how can we mobilize these assets to promote the best possible delivery of health care? We must study the issues, develop positions, decide in which political settings to take a stand, understand how the legislative process works, organize for success, and then lobby for our causes in both the federal and state legislatures.

REFERENCES

1. Mason DJ and Talbot SW: Political action handbook for nurses, Menlo Park, Calif, 1985, Addison-Wesley Publishing Co.
2. Walsh D: Personal communication, August 1988.
3. Richardson D: Personal communication, April 1989.
4. Smith-Callahan D: Personal communication, April 1989.
5. Barnett P: Personal communication, April 1989.

Chapter 8

THE ROLE OF PACs

In the 18 years since the establishment of nursing's first political action committees (PACs), nursing has become a visible and potent political force. PACs have gained influence for nurses both on Capitol Hill and in state legislatures. The growth of nursing PACs reflects nursing's increasing sophistication in the political arena. While PACs represent only part of the story, they have made a difference for nursing.

By 1986 the ANA/PAC ranked eightieth out of 4,200 PACs in terms of money given to federal candidates. Although this ranking indicates a degree of success, we must note that in the same year the American Medical Association's PAC (AMPAC, with its state affiliates known as AMA/PACs) ranked second, and the American Hospital Association's PAC (AHA/PAC) ranked sixty-seventh.[1] In 1988 the ANA/PAC contributed approximately $300,000 to the campaigns of 303 candidates running for Congress.[2] In contrast, the AM/PAC contributed $5,385,951, and the AHA/PAC contributed $513,996.[3]

PACs solicit voluntary contributions from the members of their parent organizations. Their governing boards then distribute the money to political campaigns. The purpose of PACs is to elect to public office persons friendly to the committees' positions and to be in a position to influence these persons once they are elected.

While one cannot say that PAC dollars actually buy influence, they do facilitate access to the elected officials who have received the money. Legislators have rigid constraints on their time. They are simply more likely to make themselves available to talk with persons associated with the PACs that have contributed to their campaigns than to groups or individuals who have not.

PACs are a relatively new phenomenon, yet there are now PACs to support almost every special interest and to promote every political philosophy. PACs have been established by labor unions, corporations, trade associations, cooperatives, business groups (such as realtors and automobile dealers), and professionals (such as doctors, teachers, and nurses).

PACs are also organized along ideologic lines by environmentalists, peace advocates, and groups with purely liberal or conservative agendas. PAC funds by law may be solicited only from members of the parent organization represented by the PAC, although friends of the organization may voluntarily contribute. These funds are kept separate from dues. They are used to finance political campaigns and may be used in most situations for political education, if this purpose was made clear during solicitation.

Historically, the development of PACs as a major device for campaign funding grew out of election-reform laws passed in the early 1970s. At that time there was public outcry for reform of the existing system of campaign financing—one many perceived as unfair. Federal legislators sought ways to limit the influence of the large contributions made by both individuals and organizations, to make the source of campaign funding a matter of public record, and to develop a system of public financing for presidential and congressional campaigns.

Through amendments to the Federal Election Campaign Act enacted in 1974, Congress made major changes in the laws governing the financing of presidential campaigns. It limited the size of individual campaign contributions, capped overall expenditures, and initiated public funding for presidential campaigns through the dollar check off on federal income-tax forms.[4]

The unwillingness of Congress to set up a similar public source of campaign funds for races for the House and Senate opened the door to a bigger role for PACs. The rapidly escalating costs of political campaigns had made old-fashioned fund-raising methods, such as picnics and gifts from a few wealthy donors, inadequate. By 1986 the average cost of winning a seat in the House was $355,000, for the Senate, $3,099,544.[1] PAC contributions have become the easiest way for politicians to raise substantial amounts of money. From 1977 to 1978 PACs contributed $34 million to congressional candidates. From 1987 to 1988 they contributed more than $151 million.[5]

NURSING'S FIRST PACs

In spite of their lobbying efforts at both the state and federal levels, nursing leaders in the early 1970s were having difficulty getting legislation critical to the profession passed. They found many nurses reluctant to become involved in politics and were hampered by a lack of funds to hire staff to supply the information legislators needed.

In July 1971 Rachel Rotkovitch, then Director of Nursing at Long Island Jewish Hospital, and June Rothberg, Dean of Adelphi University School of Nursing, met with a small group of nurses from their area. These nurses were interested in developing the clout necessary to influence the legislative and executive decisions affecting them. Influenced by the women's movement, the group believed that nurses can and must become involved in the political arena. They knew that AMPAC, formed in the early 1960s, had enhanced that association's power on Capitol Hill. The group concluded that nurses should be educated and then mobilized for political action.

They invited Veronica Driscoll and Cathryne Welch of the New York State Nurses' Association (NYSNA) to attend their second meeting in October 1971. While recognizing the importance of collaboration with established nursing organizations, the group decided to organize and incorporate independently of the

NYSNA or the ANA. In doing so, the group founded the first national organization committed to promoting nursing's agenda in the political arena, called Nurses for Political Action (NPA). Members of the committee starting the organization, in an extraordinary demonstration of their commitment to the new association, voted to back it personally with the needed "start-up" money. Each member agreed to lend the new organization $1,000, with the understanding that the loan would be repaid without interest if and when contributions exceeded the first year's operating expenses.[6]

About the same time, the California Nurses' Association established a PAC. Similar, legally separate committees were established later that year in connection with SNAs in Colorado, Minnesota, and Washington.[7]

By 1972 leaders of both the NPA and ANA recognized the need to work together. NPA leaders were interested in supplementing the ANA's legislative activities, and ANA leaders wanted to tap NPA enthusiasm and commitment. Representatives from the two groups met on January 17, 1973 for the first of several meetings. The ANA Board of Directors established an ad hoc committee to look into the possibility of joining forces with the NPA. The committee met on September 6, 1973, in Kansas City, Missouri, with representatives from those SNAs with established PACs serving as resource persons.

The committee recommended that the ANA establish a "carefully structured nonpartisan political action unit" guided by the association's positions, policies, and platform. On the basis of these recommendations the ANA Board of Directors established the Nurses' Coalition for Action in Politics (N-CAP), contributed $50,000 toward initial operating expenses, sought legal counsel, and set about organizing N-CAP as its PAC. The PAC's formation was then announced at the June 1974 ANA convention.

N-CAP's purposes included:
- Education of nurses on relevant political issues,
- Assistance to nurses in carrying out their civic responsibilities and organizing effective action in the political arena, and
- Raising of funds to contribute to candidates for public office who have demonstrated or indicated supportive positions on issues of importance to nurses and health care.

NPA leaders had achieved what they set out to do: to initiate a strong national nursing PAC. N-CAP had a solid beginning, so the NPA Board of Directors met on January 26, 1976, and voted to disband. To facilitate easier identification of the PAC and its parent organization, the 1985 ANA House of Delegates voted to change the PAC's name to ANA/PAC, a change that took effect in 1986.

HOW PACs ARE ORGANIZED

Federal laws govern the establishment of national PACs, and state laws (which vary from one state to another) govern PACs organized at that level. Information regarding these laws can be obtained from the national or state election commission. Even with this information, a group considering forming a PAC must seek legal counsel. Appropriate bylaws or memorandums of understanding must be in place. Officers must be elected, committees formed, contributions solicited, and a careful accounting system set up.

It should be clear that PACs do not set priorities or establish general policy for their parent organizations. PACs do no direct lobbying. By law their function is to raise money and provide financial and other support for candidates of their choice, especially those candidates who support the legislative goals of the PACs' parent organizations.

Headquarters of ANA/PAC are at the Washington, D.C., office of the ANA. A Congressional District Coordinator (CDC) Network, organized under the ANA Department of Political Education, serves as a liaison between the PAC's Board of Directors and the field. The PAC's goal is to have at least one CDC in every one of the 435 congressional districts.

HOW ANA/PAC'S CDCs FUNCTION

CDCs' most important job is to organize nurses to help elect ANA/PAC-endorsed candidates. CDCs represent the PAC in the field, keep in touch with candidates and potential candidates and their organizations, provide information and advice relevant to the endorsement process to the ANA/PAC board, work in endorsed candidates' campaigns, and serve as resource persons to candidates on health-related issues during the campaign—and after, if the candidate is elected.

Donna Mahrenholz and Kathleen White shared the responsibilities of CDC in the 1986 Maryland campaign in which Congresswoman Barbara Mikulski ran for the U.S. Senate. As ANA/PAC representatives they were invited to a strategy session for Mikulski campaign workers one Sunday afternoon in the spring. Mahrenholz says:

> A number of types of activities were discussed—phone banks, fund-raisers, a booth at the state fair, and standing on street corners with Mikulski signs.
> We decided to pick and choose the tasks we would accept. We wanted to assist the campaign, but we also looked on this as an opportunity for positive image-making for nurses. In accepting tasks, we tried to be sensitive to what we thought nurses would be comfortable doing. As an example, we didn't think most nurses would want to stand on street corners holding signs, so we just said no to that.
> We chose jobs in which we believed nursing would have an impact. When requests were made, we trimmed them down—and then always produced more than we'd agreed to do. Rather than promising more than we could deliver, we delivered more than we promised. For instance, the campaign committee asked us to do 10 fund-raisers. We agreed to do five—and then did eight. This reinforced the idea that nurses are capable and dependable.

SNA/PACs are organized in a manner similar to the ANA/PAC's organization. A Board of Directors is elected and, depending on the number of active members in the PAC, committees for endorsements and fund-raising may be formed. The state is divided geographically, often in the same way DNAs are divided. At least one nurse represents each district. This representative's responsibilities to the SNA/PAC parallel those of the CDC to the ANA/PAC.

ENDORSEMENTS AND HOW THEY ARE MADE

Endorsements are the critical element of PAC activity. Through them an association makes a statement about its position on issues with which it is concerned. Each PAC has a policy on endorsement of candidates, and each one has an endorsement committee, which may include some or all of the members of the board of directors. For more information, ask your SNA/PAC to send you a copy of its endorsement guidelines.

Endorsements are made on the basis of answers to questionnaires, personal interviews, voting records of incumbents, information from the field about candidates' accessibility to nurses and support for nursing positions, and evaluations from the association's lobbyist.

Questionnaires

Questionnaires must be carefully crafted so that responses reflect the candidate's positions accurately. Then a system for evaluation of these responses must be devised. (A questionnaire used in 1986 by the Maryland Nurses' Association PAC is shown on pp. 118-119 as an example.)

Questionnaires actually educate candidates on the organization's positions. Conscientious legislators want to know where organizations representing large numbers of potential voters stand on issues. When the MNA/PAC sent out its first questionnaire, my colleagues in the state legislature called me for help. They wanted to know what nursing's positions were on the issues raised in the questionnaire. I set up several little conferences to share information. These sessions proved to be a wonderful way to educate my colleagues on issues of importance to nursing, to answer questions, and to promote substantive dialog.

For candidates, questionnaires present problems as well as opportunities. Answering them thoughtfully requires time, and each election brings more of them. To give you an idea of the magnitude of the task, I received 50 questionnaires the year I ran for the Maryland Senate (1986).

Like those sent out by newspapers, questionnaires sent out by PACs frequently require 45-word answers to complex questions. Extra words are simply cut. This conciseness requirement presents candidates with the difficult task of crafting every answer into what amounts to a "sound bite" (the technique used by television producers to limit complicated messages to 30-second segments).

When I ran for office the first time, I found these questionnaires overwhelming. Many of the questions dealt with issues on which I had no expertise at that time, so I asked incumbents if the issues had been addressed in previous legislative sessions and if the issues were important to the community at large or just to the group asking the question. Members of my political party, especially the incumbents, gave me valuable assistance.

No politician wants to be locked into positions he or she may want to change later. Therefore, I added a qualifying note to every questionnaire saying that my answers were based on current knowledge but that I reserved the right to change my opinion based on new information.

Interviews

Personal interviews with candidates conducted by members of the PAC's endorsement committee help PACs assess candidates' support for the organization's political agenda. These sessions also offer opportunities to educate candidates on nursing positions.

Mahrenholz and White cochaired the committee that interviewed most of Maryland's congressional candidates in 1986. (The politically experienced nurses who lived in Annapolis, our state capital, conducted interviews with candidates from their districts.) Mahrenholz has strong ideas on how these interviews should be conducted:

> First of all, insist that candidates are interviewed on nursing's turf. This puts the candidate in the position of coming to us. It gives nurses more control over the interview. We invited candidates to meet our committee at MNA headquarters. While one candidate was reluctant, when it was made clear to her campaign staff that we would not even consider endorsing her unless she came to us, she came.
> As the most experienced person in our group, I opened the interview by saying, "If we endorse you, we can help you. This is what we can do. We would like to know what you would want from us." We had a list of questions to which we wanted answers from the candidates. I opened the questioning, and then other nurses joined in. I think it is very important for nurses just entering political work to have visible role models. It is one thing to tell inexperienced people what should be done, but it is far more valuable to show them.[8]

It is helpful if the same team of questioners interviews candidates for the same office. At the close of the interview, the candidate should be told when the committee will make its decision.

How do candidates prepare for these interviews? The first time I ran for office, a business group asked for an interview. I called the group's office and asked the organization to send to me any written information it had about its organizational structure, the issues about which members were concerned, and the names of persons on its PAC board.

I familiarized myself with all of the material the group sent and asked incumbents for more information about the group. By the time of the interview, I felt nervous but comfortable that I had prepared for the session as well as I could have. The interview was difficult, but the interviewers complimented me on my understanding of the issues, especially since I was not an incumbent. My research paid off, for 2 weeks later I was informed that I had won the group's endorsement, which brought campaign contributions, volunteers for my campaign, and a mailing from them to their membership.

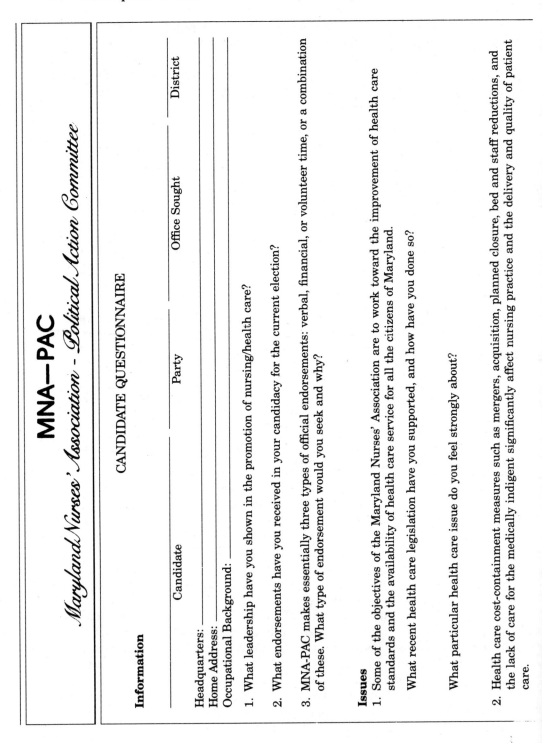

MNA—PAC

Maryland Nurses' Association - Political Action Committee

CANDIDATE QUESTIONNAIRE

Information

Candidate	Party	Office Sought	District

Headquarters: _____

Home Address: _____

Occupational Background: _____

1. What leadership have you shown in the promotion of nursing/health care?

2. What endorsements have you received in your candidacy for the current election?

3. MNA-PAC makes essentially three types of official endorsements: verbal, financial, or volunteer time, or a combination of these. What type of endorsement would you seek and why?

Issues

1. Some of the objectives of the Maryland Nurses' Association are to work toward the improvement of health care standards and the availability of health care service for all the citizens of Maryland.

   What recent health care legislation have you supported, and how have you done so?

   What particular health care issue do you feel strongly about?

2. Health care cost-containment measures such as mergers, acquisition, planned closure, bed and staff reductions, and the lack of care for the medically indigent significantly affect nursing practice and the delivery and quality of patient care.

How have you been involved in cost-containment initiatives?

What specific measures would you propose to address cost-containment dilemmas?

3. In what ways would you ensure the active involvement of the nursing profession in the policy development and decision making related to health care issues?

Specifically, to which task force or committee will you appoint nurses?

4. The Maryland Nurses' Association is concerned with pay equity for nurses throughout the state of Maryland. In what way would you support the organization's endeavor to achieve pay equity?

5. What is your position on the following health care issues facing your constituency?

a) Requirements for smoke-free areas in public facilities, such as restaurants, public buildings, meeting places, etc.

b) Criminal-record checks for (1) child care workers and (2) elder-care workers.

QUESTIONNAIRES MUST BE RECEIVED BY JULY 18, 1986 AT 5 PM TO BE CONSIDERED FOR AN ENDORSEMENT.

Signature of Candidate _____

5820 Southwestern Blvd. Baltimore, Maryland 21227

801-242-7800

Most politicians like interviews because they provide opportunities to get across through body language and voice inflection the messages that don't come through in written form.

THE INCUMBENT'S ADVANTAGE

In any political race incumbents have real advantages. They are known figures. Their day-to-day performance of their duties keeps them in the public eye. There usually has to be a good reason for an incumbent to be unseated. PAC boards know that voters consistently reelect incumbents if they have provided their constituents with appropriate services and have represented them well. At the federal level the number of reelected incumbents is startling. In 1988, 99% of the incumbents in the House of Representatives who ran for reelection won, and approximately 90% of incumbent senators running for reelection were returned to office.[9]

As PACs become increasingly interested in the influence their contributions will buy after elections, more of their money goes to likely winners. Incumbents running for Congress in 1988 received more than 74% of PAC money,[5] greatly compounding the problems of their political challengers (Fig. 8-1). But in some elections PACs hedge their contributions by giving to the campaigns of opposing candidates, assuring themselves of influence over whoever wins.

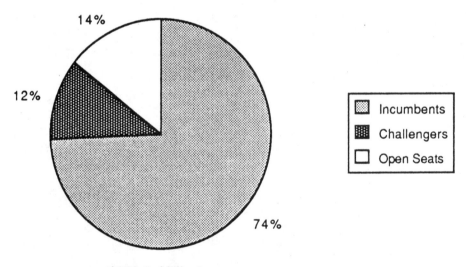

14%

12%

74%

	Incumbents
	Challengers
	Open Seats

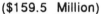

($159.5 Million)

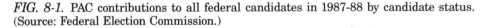

FIG. 8-1. PAC contributions to all federal candidates in 1987-88 by candidate status. (Source: Federal Election Commission.)

Although PACs are less influential at the state than the federal level, incumbents holding state offices still have a distinct advantage. In my first campaign for the Maryland House of Delegates, fundraising was difficult and painful. Members of the local business community—substantial contributors to local campaigns—made certain assumptions about me as a newcomer. They believed that I would not be an active supporter of their issues, based on my community activities and my status as a registered nurse. That year, I received a negligible amount of money from them and the PACs.

However, when I ran for reelection 4 years later, the business community contributed to my campaign. Its members had found that they could work with me. Contributions from organized special-interest groups increased. Lobbyists believed that I would become an increasingly influential member of the House of Delegates and encouraged their PACs to support me.

By the time I ran for reelection the third time, I was moving into a leadership position in the House of Delegates. PACs that had not supported my past campaigns began to contribute. These experiences confirmed my conviction that incumbency is the greatest factor in a candidate's ability to raise money.

OPEN RACES

Open races, those in which no incumbent is running, present special opportunities for both candidates and PACs. These races are usually hotly contested. When PACs consider contributing to candidates in these contests, they can assume that the winner has an excellent chance of being returned to office election after election.

Sometimes when there is an open race, a PAC may be faced with a difficult decision. The ANA/PAC was confronted with such a decision when it looked at the open race for a Maryland seat in the U.S. Senate in 1986. Republican Senator Charles Mathias retired that year. The strong possibility of capturing his seat created a free-for-all in Maryland's Democratic Party. Democrats outnumber Republicans significantly in voter registration in Maryland, giving them an important advantage. In this case the primary became more interesting than the general election because three well-qualified candidates entered the race for the Democratic nomination.

One of them was Governor Harry Hughes, a popular politician who had always given verbal support to nursing but had developed no administrative initiatives to benefit the profession.

A second candidate was Congressman Michael Barnes, from Montgomery County. He voted favorably on nursing issues and was a "favorite son" of nurses in our district. He served on both the Budget and Foreign Affairs committees on Capitol Hill and had concentrated on Latin American foreign policy.

The third candidate was Congresswoman Barbara Mikulski, from Baltimore. A former social worker, she had demonstrated interest in nursing issues. She had frequently been in touch with me on nursing matters and, where possible, had used my bills as models for similar legislation in Congress. Her committee assignments put her in positions to influence health policy.

ANA/PAC members asked themselves: "Who had the better chance?" and "Who, if elected, would be in the best position to help nursing?" The committee concluded that Mikulski was the answer to both questions. It gave her a "high-priority" endorsement before the primary, contributed financially to her campaign, and began to mobilize Maryland nurses to work for her election.

THE ENDORSEMENT ITSELF

When all data are in, including the recommendations of the association's lobbyist, the PAC's endorsement committee looks first at incumbents running for reelection. It takes into consideration how influential the candidate is on health matters. Does he or she serve on a committee that deals with this kind of legislation? Does he or she have a leadership position? In short, who would help nursing most? The committee may vote to endorse the incumbent and then follow up with financial and other means of support for the campaign.

Then the committee looks at challengers—particularly if they are mounting campaigns against incumbents who have been unfriendly to nursing. If the candidate seems particularly worthy of support, the committee may decide not only to endorse him or her but also to contribute extra money to the campaign, realizing that the candidate's need is greater.

Nursing PACs tend to support female candidates when possible. And candidates who are nurses are almost always singled out for enthusiastic endorsements and substantial support.

SNA ENDORSEMENTS

For SNA/PACs, making endorsements can be problematic because of the number of contests and the limited supply of available workers. There are many exceptions because state constitutions vary, but Senate terms typically last 4 years, and terms in the lower house most commonly last 2 years. During state elections, therefore, SNA/PACs—usually with fewer people to do the work—are faced with making endorsements from among a large number of candidates. For example, in the Maryland General Assembly (an exception to the above generalization about terms of offices) both Senators and Delegates serve 4-year terms. These terms are not staggered, so during the quadrennial elections (except for the few in which an incumbent has no challenger) all 188 seats are contested.

Barbara Hanley, RN, PhD, and Katie Berry cochaired the MNA/PAC in 1986. Hanley says:

> At that time the PAC was faced with an incredible number of legislators pressing us for our endorsements. We only considered candidates who had returned our questionnaire. Some 300 did. The endorsement process we had used in 1982, in

which we handled data manually and the committee worked in all-night sessions, proved to be inadequate.

We are now developing a computerized list of legislators that can be kept up-to-date on an ongoing basis. We will count on nurses in each MNA district to gather information on legislators' voting records, accessibility, and evidenced support for nursing. This, we believe, will help us at endorsement time and also encourage regular communication between nurses and legislators.

We have found that nurses are respected and trusted. Our endorsements are deemed valuable. We must find ways in our endorsement process to allow early endorsements of our known friends.[10]

FUNDRAISING

Besides endorsing them, PACs also support candidates by contributing financially to their campaigns. Nursing PACs have adopted some inventive ways to raise funds. ANA/PAC has had increasing success in raising money. At the 1988 ANA convention, held in Louisville, Kentucky, the PAC raised $39,000 in a "challenge" that lasted approximately 10 minutes.[11] (This technique is also used successfully at SNA conventions or at any event at which large numbers of politically aware nurses gather.) Hanley describes the fundraising method:

Before the event the leader has several friends planted in the audience. The "challenge" is announced as a fundraising event for the PAC. The first "friend" raises her hand or stands and may say, "I am a nursing educator and believe that nursing goals can be furthered through political action. The PAC, by endorsing candidates and contributing to their campaigns, ensures our influence with elected officials. I will donate $25 to the PAC, and challenge other nursing educators to do so." A second nursing educator rises and says, "I accept the challenge and will donate $30. Will others of our colleagues join us?" And the challenge continues.

The same scenario is repeated with staff nurses, administrators, psychiatric nurses, and others. When enthusiasm is high, a large amount of money can be collected quickly.[10]

A second event at the 1988 ANA convention raised an additional $2,900 for the ANA/PAC. A silent auction for political items was set up in an exhibit hall. Nurses could place written bids on items such as a trip to Washington, D.C., lunch with Florida Representative Claude Pepper (now deceased), an ANA "Proud to Care" poster autographed by 1984 Democratic Vice-Presidential candidate Geraldine Ferraro, and a copy of the Community Nursing Organization bill, autographed by its sponsor, Missouri Congressman Richard Gephardt. Such a fund-raiser could be attempted on a smaller scale in other places.

In an effort to encourage larger contributions, the ANA/PAC established in 1988 a $100 Club for nurses who had contributed that amount or more to the PAC. Challenges to join the club stimulated generous contributions at the "challenge" fund-raiser. Members of the $100 Club were given buttons and treated to a special reception at the convention.

In 1986 "Nurses for Mikulski" sponsored a "No-come party." They included a tea bag with their request for campaign funds, which read: "Have tea with

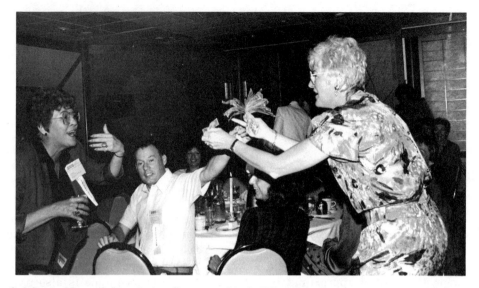

California Nurses' Association Secretary Linda Kinrade collects money at a 1987 fundraiser for the CNA/PAC, the California Nurses Foundation, and the CNA scholarship program. (From The California Nurse 83:9, 1987. Photo by Maureen Anderson.)

Barbara Mikulski in the comfort of your own home. Please send us $2." Busy people found this an appealing approach.

At the 1987 California Nurses' Association convention, $1,500 was raised in one evening to benefit the CNA/PAC, the California Nurses Foundation, and the CNA's scholarship program. Organizers planned a "Fun-raiser, dinner, and talent show," in which nurses paid $25 to perform, and others paid to get them off stage. Officers of the CNA Board of Directors, the PAC, and CNA structural units presented their own versions of popular favorites, such as "I Left My Heart in San Francisco," "Born in the CNA" (a takeoff on "Born in the USA"), and "California Girl."[12]

Both ANA/PAC and some SNA/PACs have solicited PAC contributions when billing for annual dues. More recently, several SNAs have introduced "dues designation" or "negative dues checkoff" as a way to fund their PACs. In these states SNA bylaws specify that a specific amount, for example, $5, of each member's dues be deposited in the SNA/PAC fund but that individuals may choose to have the money reallocated in some specific way. For example, in California, Illinois, and Florida, SNA members wishing not to contribute to the PAC may request that their money go into the General Fund. Billing for dues must clearly identify the PAC contribution as an extra fund. It must be separated as a contribution, and the SNA member must be given the option of a refund or reallocation of the money. SNAs that have been able to institute this

NURSES CARE!

Nurses care about the health care system.

Nurses believe costs can be controlled by increasing competition in the health care industry; by reducing the artificial restraints which prevent nurses from providing care they are qualified to give.

Nurses are becoming a powerful political force, demanding full support for quality health care.

Nurses not only vote but also volunteer to work for the candidates they support.

NURSES ARE EVEN MORE POWERFUL IN POLITICS BECAUSE OF ANA-PAC: THE POLITICAL CAMPAIGN FUND OF THE AMERICAN NURSES' ASSOCIATION.

ANA-PAC's power comes from thousands of nurses, pooling their financial contributions to support political candidates who will work for a strong health care system.

YOUR $25 ADDS UP!

In the 1986 election, ANA-PAC gave $300,000 to candidates who will stand up for a strong health-care system.

And of all the candidates we endorsed, 90% won election to the House or Senate!

Thousands of State Nurses' Association members like you include their ANA-PAC contributions along with their membership renewal forms.

Right now, as you renew your membership dues, you can "write in" a contribution to ANA-PAC on your membership renewal form, and include your contribution of $25 with your dues payment.

PUT YOUR $25 WHERE IT WILL DO THE MOST GOOD.

When you contribute $25 to ANA-PAC, your contribution goes into the campaigns of political candidates who support a strong health care system. Your $25 contribution is put to work in a political campaign.

And ANA-PAC assures that your dollars go where they will do the most good.

Our Board of Trustees reviews the record of each candidate for the U.S. Senate and House of Representatives. We talk to nurses back home. We gather information on every Congressional race in the country. Then we decide which candidates deserve our endorsement, and which need the special help of a contribution.

GIFTS OF LEADERSHIP: THE ANA-PAC "$100 Club"

ANA-PAC supporters who contribute $100 or more are welcomed to the ANA-PAC "$100 Club." Members of the "$100 Club" will receive a special "$100 Club" Pin to acknowledge their special generosity.

Your contribution of $100 or more will give nurses a more powerful voice in Washington, where government decisions shape so much of our professional lives.

If you are one of the fortunate members who can make a substantial contribution . . . we urge you to take the lead as a member of ANA-PAC'S "$100 Club."

TWO WAYS TO CONTRIBUTE TO ANA-PAC . . .

1. When you renew with SNA/ANA, just write in the amount of your ANA-PAC contribution and add that amount to your dues check.

2. Or you can make a contribution at any time with the coupon attached to this flyer. Just fill in the coupon and mail it with your check to ANA-PAC, 1101 14th Street, NW, Washington, DC 20005.

When you contribute $25, $50, $100 — or any amount you choose — you are helping to elect Senators and Representatives who will defend and strengthen the American health care system.

Your $25 contribution supports a strong health-care system.

Example of ANA/PAC's fundraising brochure, which allowed PAC contributions to be made along with dues payments. Courtesy American Nurses' Association.

method of PAC funding have found it very effective. Such funding practices are subject to state laws and, therefore, vary from state to state. Legal counsel is a prerequisite to the introduction of amendments to an SNA's bylaws that create such a funding method.

For additional ideas about fundraising see "Tips for PAC fundraising" (Appendix F).

HOW ARE CONTRIBUTIONS ALLOCATED?

PAC boards decide how contributions will be allocated. SNA/PACs have less money to distribute than the national PAC. Often, the problem is how to use it wisely. For example, in the 1986 election, before the MNA's adoption of dues designation as a method of funding its PAC, the MNA/PAC had only $1,800 to contribute to the large number of candidates it endorsed. Its board decided to spend $150 to purchase a set of name and address labels from the Maryland Board of Nursing for all the registered nurses in the state.

The labels were arranged according to zip codes, so it was possible for committee members to divide the labels according to legislative districts by comparing addresses with street maps. Then appropriate labels were given to endorsed candidates in each district. The balance of the PAC funds was divided evenly among the four nurses running for seats in the House of Delegates. The MNA/PAC board's allocations were a creative way to use limited funds.

BEYOND MONEY: OTHER WAYS TO SUPPORT A CANDIDATE

Mailing labels, like those previously described, are a valuable campaign contribution that is relatively inexpensive for the PAC. The candidate can use these labels to target nurses with relevant campaign literature. (For more information about targeted campaign materials, see Chapter 10.)

The support and involvement of capable, efficient campaign workers are nursing's most valuable contribution to many campaigns. These nurses write issue papers and perform the "nitty-gritty" tasks of any campaign, including folding literature, stuffing envelopes, staffing telephone banks, walking with candidates in neighborhoods, and distributing campaign materials door-to-door or in public places. No matter what the activity, when nurses campaign, they should identify themselves as nurses.

Mahrenholz believes that nurses should have two questions in mind when they plan efforts to assist candidates: What can we do for the candidate? And how can we gain maximum positive visibility for nurses? How did "Nurses for [Barbara] Mikulski" accomplish both of these goals in 1986? Mahrenholz says:

> Rather than have nurses drift in and out of Mikulski headquarters at unscheduled times, we decided to present ourselves as a group, so that our contribution would be easily recognized. We sponsored five "Nurses' Nights" on the Mikulski telephone bank. On each of those evenings, 10 or 12 nurses took over all of the phones, calling voters to ask them to vote for Mikulski. The nurses came at 6 PM and went right to work. Campaign managers said that the nurses made more calls than any other group. It was an impressive show of nurse power.
>
> Wherever nurses worked in the campaign, they wore "Nurses for Mikulski" buttons, thereby making their identity clear.[8]

Telephone banks have become an important part of political campaigns. Occasionally, a nurse is asked to organize one. Such was the case in 1988 when Denise Kishel, as ANA/PAC coordinator for the presidential campaign in Maryland, was requested to organize phone calls to more than 3,000 MNA members to remind them of the PAC's endorsement and to urge them to vote.

How did Kishel organize this enormous task? She divided the list of MNA members by district associations and parceled out the lists to PAC representatives in each district. She concluded that local calls must be made from central locations in each district and that the task would be more efficiently done by groups of nurses working together. Her problem was to find facilities in which there were several phones, so that a number of nurses could make calls at one time. Tapping a variety of possibilities, she found appropriate office spaces, arranged dates, and recruited nurses. "The hours between 5 PM and 9 PM have proven to be the best time to reach people at home," she says.[13]

Ten nurses from my district made calls from the nearby ANA headquarters in Washington one evening after the office closed. Nurses in neighboring Prince George's County telephoned from the local community college. Baltimore nurses called from the MNA offices. By organizing the effort into time blocks and dividing the work, the task was accomplished with a minimum of effort. Once again, people were impressed with nursing's delivery on its commitment. A side benefit for the nurses was the spirit of camaraderie that developed as they worked together.

USING THE MEDIA

PAC endorsements offer public relations opportunities for both candidates and PACs. Press releases announcing endorsements should be distributed to both the print and electronic media. Whenever possible, photographs should accompany releases. Remember that local newspapers and radio and television stations are more likely to use this information. Candidates frequently list the organizations that endorse them when they talk with the press. These acknowledgments help both the candidate and the endorsing PACs.

Members of nursing associations must be kept informed. State and district newsletters must publicize endorsements and, when possible, carry feature and news stories about favored candidates. Copies of these publications should be sent to candidates to reinforce their awareness of what the association is doing to promote their campaigns. (For more information on how to gain maximum exposure from the news media, review Chapter 5.)

BENEFITS

There are many personal satisfactions to be gained from working in an election campaign. They include the feeling of being a player in our participatory democracy and the pleasures of building associations with like-minded people. When candidates endorsed by nursing PACs win, many benefits accrue to the profession. During the campaign, nurses will have established their ability to deliver results after making a commitment. Positive relationships between nurses and elected officials will have been formed. Politicians will know they can work with us. So when our candidates win, nurses must not shy or fade away. Nurses can continue to be valuable to officeholders by serving as resource people on health care matters. Experts in the nursing profession should analyze health care budgets and lobby for appropriate changes when they are necessary.

Nursing organizations should forward to the person in office lists of members who could serve on boards or commissions, with the expectation that the elected official will at least consider their recommendations. Every SNA should establish a talent bank, so that when there is a vacancy on one of these boards or commissions, the SNA has a name to submit. And nurses can reinforce positive relationships with elected officials whom they have endorsed by asking them to speak at nursing conventions and forums.

PAC REFORM: A QUESTION

PACs offer contributors of small amounts an opportunity to increase the effect of the money they give to political campaigns. Through PACs, like-minded citizens pool their contributions and direct their resources toward the election of candidates who support their group's special interests. A PAC may give up to $5,000 per election to a candidate and may give to as many candidates as it chooses. But the law requires timely and accurate reporting of contributions and other spending.

Most politically aware people agree that with the proliferation of PACs more people than ever are making contributions to political campaigns. A contribution of even a small amount of money heightens the donor's interest in a contest. The experience has been likened to betting on a horse race: By placing even a $2 bet, you have a stake in the outcome.

In addition to raising funds and distributing them to candidates for election, PACs emphasize political education and grass-roots activism. During a period when civics lessons are often neglected in schools, PAC efforts to educate members about the workings of the government and to encourage their participation in the political process are real contributions to the public good.

What troubles some people about PACs is what seems to be the increased stridency of special-interest groups and what is perceived to be the potentially corrupting influence of the large amounts of money they contribute.

PAC money has become an increasingly attractive way to finance political campaigns. Critics worry that the recipients of this money are put in a position to be unfairly influenced when they vote on an issue on which the PAC holds a strong position. Contributing to the controversy is the increasing cost of political campaigns. For example, the $355,000 average cost in 1986 of winning campaigns for the U.S. House of Representatives required incumbents to raise approximately $15,000 every month during their 2-year terms.

The average cost of winning a 1986 Senate campaign was more than $3 million; thus U.S. Senators needed to raise approximately $10,000 per week during their 6 years in office. (We will talk about the cost of campaigns for state legislatures in Chapter 10.)

While individual contributors provide the bulk of campaign money for congressional races, contributions from PACs make up increasingly high percentages of politicians' campaign funds. There is no question that PAC money gives incumbents the advantage. Our founding fathers envisioned the House of Representatives as the chamber most responsive to the people, but it seems that once elected, a representative can hold the seat as long as he or she is interested.

Loopholes in present laws allow PACs and individuals to funnel money that is not accounted for into election campaigns. Two of these loopholes are of special note. One is "soft money," gifts that can go to political parties but not to candidates. These contributions, in undisclosed amounts, are supposedly confined to "party-building" activities at the state and local levels. But evidence suggests that this money is in fact spent in connection with the election campaigns of candidates for federal offices.

A second loophole allows PACs and individuals to make unlimited contributions on behalf of or in opposition to a candidate, as long as it is done "independently," that is, without coordination or consultation with the candidate. This loophole has been at least partly responsible for a disturbing development: the intrusion of out-of-state PAC money into local races. Such was the case in 1980, when the National Conservative Political Action Committee (NCPAC) launched an aggressive television campaign to unseat six U.S. Senators whom they judged to be liberal. Four of the targeted Senators—George McGovern (D-S.D.), John Culver (D-Iowa), Frank Church (D-Idaho), and Birch Bayh (D-Ind.)—went down in defeat. Many people believe that NCPAC's effort—financed by a well-heeled national rather than local group—was a major contributing factor.[1]

Two years later, NCPAC mounted an expensive campaign to defeat Maryland's Democratic Senator Paul Sarbanes. Newspaper editorials, letters to the editor, and spokespersons for citizen's groups reflected the anger that Maryland residents felt at this outside interference in the politics of our state. Senator Sarbanes was a respected, popular legislator. Chances are strong that he would have been reelected anyway, but many people believe that backlash against NCPAC's intrusion also may have contributed to the substantial majority with which Senator Sarbanes was returned to office.

Some people worry that important groups of the electorate are not represented by PACs. Senator Robert Dole (R-Kan.) has said, "There aren't any poor PACs or food stamp PACs or nutrition PACs or Medicare PACs."[14] Former Senator Gary Hart (D-Colo.) has commented that there is no well-heeled PAC representing the interests of the average citizen, "the voter who has no special interest beyond low taxes, an efficient government, an honorable Congress, and a humane society."[4] But in spite of the absence of PACs to push for them, food stamps, nutrition, and Medicare programs exist because a large segment of the electorate supports services for vulnerable populations.

Both Democratic and Republican legislators, as well as many citizens' groups (such as Common Cause), call for reforms in campaign financing. In 1985 senators with disparate political philosophies, such as Barry Goldwater (R-

Ariz.) and David Boren (D-Okla.), joined forces to sponsor a bill that would have limited the amount of PAC money a congressional candidate could receive. The Senate passed it with a vote of 69-30, but the initiative went no further.[1] Many people call for reform, but at the time of this writing, Congress had not come to terms with the problem.

In spite of the concerns about them, the reality is that PACs are an important part of today's political system. Nursing PACs increase the profession's visibility and effectiveness on Capitol Hill and in state legislatures. PAC contributions virtually guarantee nurses access to legislators when issues important to the profession are under discussion.

Nursing PAC leaders urge members to support endorsed candidates. It is in the interest of the PAC—and nursing—to make endorsements. Leaders know that nurses are citizens first and PAC supporters second. As citizens they will vote according to their consciences, usually on the basis of more than one issue. It is possible with a clear conscience to support a PAC with campaign contributions for the benefit of nursing and to vote independently.

With the exception of the years between 1982 and 1985, Barbara Curtis has been a member of the ANA/PAC Board of Directors since its inception. She says:

> During that time I have seen the whole profession move from a state of naiveté to quite a high level of political sophistication. We have seen a tremendous increase in nurses' level of involvement in the political arena. They now see the relationship between legislation and the health care system in which they practice. They understand that our PACs help elect people sympathetic to our positions and facilitate access to them once they are in office.[15]

The rapid growth of nursing PACs and nurses' ability to utilize their influence to achieve health policy goals are, among others, signs that nurses have come of age in the political system. If nurses are to play the political game, we must support our PACs both with money and by participation in the campaigns of our endorsed candidates. Our work in the political field is as valuable to candidates as money. The visibility attracted by politically active nurses creates an image of nurses as a powerful political force.

REFERENCES

1. Stern PM: The best Congress money can buy, New York, 1988, Pantheon Books, Inc.
2. Ford-Roegner P: Personal communication, November 1988.
3. Miletich DM: Personal communication, February 22, 1989.
4. Wertheimer F: Campaign finance reform: the unfinished agenda, Annals, American Academy of Political and Social Science 486:88-91, July 1986.
5. Federal Election Commission: FEC finds slower growth of PAC activity during 1988 election cycle (press release), April 9, 1989, Washington, DC.
6. Mason DJ and Talbott SW: Political action handbook for nurses, Menlo Park, Calif, 1985, Addison-Wesley Publishing Co.
7. ANA/PAC: N-CAP history (fact sheet), April 1974.
8. Mahrenholz D: Personal communication, November 1988.
9. More political money (editorial), The Washington Post, November 11, 1988.

10. Hanley B: Personal communication, November 1988.
11. ANA-PAC collects $39,000, The American Nurse, July-August 1988.
12. Fun-raiser takes the cake, The California Nurse 83:9, November 1987.
13. Kishel D: Personal communication, November 1988.
14. Sabato LJ: PAC power: inside the world of political action committees, New York, 1984, WW Norton & Co, Inc.
15. Curtis B: Personal communication, November 1988.

Chapter 9

⫻ RISK TAKERS AND ROLE BREAKERS

The Chinese character for crisis combines two components, the symbols for challenge and opportunity, each of which can stand alone. The interrelationship of these three concepts became apparent to nurses in the late 1980s when acute shortages of nurses, the introduction of cost-containment regulations, and the needs of a growing population of elderly citizens created an upheaval in nursing and health care.

If somewhat intimidating, such tumultuous change is always challenging. However, with faith, vision, and hard work, most situations can be improved. Therefore, as we look for ways to solve the day-to-day crises in nursing, we must look beyond them to find the opportunities that are always inherent in major change. Resolution of the problems associated with any crisis often requires bold new ways of looking at potential solutions—as well as some educated risk-taking.

We need nurses who see our profession realistically, value it for what it is, and hold fast to their special visions of what it can become. In working to make these dreams reality, these nurses—no matter what their areas of practice—will be in the vanguard of change. Each in her or his way proves that nurses are professionals, ready and willing to assume responsibility for clients, as well as leadership roles in health care.

In this chapter we will look at stories that illustrate what nurses can do to create positive change, whether they are giving direct patient care, supporting it educationally or administratively, or operating in the larger arena of health policy. Nurses in all these fields have found within themselves the motivation to try to resolve problems and to learn the skills—frequently political—that have enabled them to make a difference. Each nurse in a different way is a risk taker and role breaker. Insomuch as these nurses inspire others, they are also role models. The following stories are typical of the stories that could be told about many other nurses across the United States. We have asked these nurses to tell their stories from their own perspectives, because each nurse has faced a different sort of challenge and each one has found a way to make a difference.

THE SECRETARY OF A STATE HEALTH DEPARTMENT

Adele Wilzack, RN, MS, has held a position in the governor's cabinet as Secretary of the Maryland Department of Health and Mental Hygiene since 1983. She is both the first woman and the first nurse to hold this powerful position. As head of the department, she oversees the work of more than 10,000 employees and is responsible for an annual budget of approximately $1 billion. How did Wilzack attain this extraordinarily influential position? And what observations would she like to share with other nurses? She says:

> Barbara Mikulski* and I became friends while attending the parochial high school in the Baltimore neighborhood in which we grew up. We have always shared the desire to make the world a better place. Barbara went into social work, and I became a nurse.
> Following graduation I worked several years at Baltimore's Mercy Hospital, the hospital where I trained.
> One day in the early 1960s while I was working on floor, Barbara came to see me. She said, "We should get involved in the War on Poverty." This program, initiated by President Lyndon Johnson, was predicated on his conviction that the poor

---

*Barbara Mikulski became a U.S. Senator from Maryland in 1986.

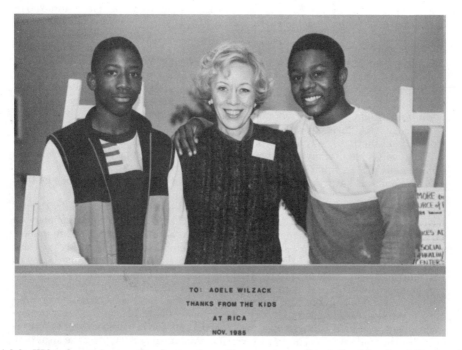

Adele Wilzack receives a thank you from the young people at the Maryland Regional Institute for Children and Adolescents.

should be involved in solving their own problems. The idea appealed to me. At the time, I was chairing a hospital committee working with aides and orderlies. I believed my experience would prove valuable in developing programs based on this premise.

As time had gone on, I had wished to be in a position to have more control over programs in which I felt I could make a difference. This seemed to present a real opportunity. With some reluctance I left the hospital.

Barbara and I organized a demonstration program in south Baltimore, in which we educated elderly members of the black community to become health aides. We taught these "friendly visitors" to do dressings, give medications, assist and assess the needs of the more elderly and infirm in their own community. The program, Operation Reason, which was originally funded for 2 years in 1965, is in existence today. To launch this program and see it sustained required more than nursing knowledge. It required understanding of city and state politics and familiarity with the influential people. I found I liked politics.

Maryland's Governor William Donald Schaefer, Barbara, and I worked together in Baltimore's city government. In 1967 Schaefer, then the mayor of Baltimore, appointed me Assistant Director, Bureau of Special Home Services in the Baltimore City Health Department. Here I was addressing the health needs of the chronically ill. In that and subsequent positions I held in Baltimore, I was increasingly involved in administration of programs targeted at providing health care for the medically indigent and the elderly.

On the basis of this experience and my growing expertise, in 1979 Governor Harry Hughes asked me to administer the state medical assistance program under the Maryland Department of Health and Mental Hygiene. The program at that time was plagued by an $80 million deficit. I went to work, made innovative changes, worked with the legislature, and slowly but surely we were able to reverse the deficit.

The governor knew and respected me. With two others, I had developed position papers for him during his campaign for governor. When the Secretary of the Department of Health and Mental Hygiene resigned in 1983, I was but one of several who were considered for the top leadership position. It became clear to me that if I wanted the position, I could not leave it to chance. I let the governor know of my interest and then mobilized support for my candidacy.

In time the governor called me into his office for what became a 3-hour interview. I told him that I would work hard, be loyal, would carry out his program, but would always give him my honest opinion. A few days later he called me back and quietly gave me the appointment.

No one was surprised when Governor Schaefer reappointed me when he took office in 1988.

When you administer a large enterprise, there are internal and external forces that affect your success. Your staff is a key. Their respect is vital. Somehow as an administrator, you must make it clear that you and they are bonded in values. Everyone in the department should feel a proprietorship in an idea. My goal has been to promote a concern for people. Within the department there must be joy in mutual success. A successful administrator creates an environment where things can happen, one where individuals can assume responsibility for themselves.

Analyzing situations and finding ways to resolve problems comes second nature to nurses. We are used to integrating things quickly. I often think my experience as a hospital float nurse was good preparation for my present work. You remember the challenge of coming to a new floor and quickly surveying the situation. Which patients will need the most care? Where are the tools with which I can do the work? Who can be counted on to help? How can we provide for the less critical needs of others on the floor? An administrator makes similar assessments and organizes the work accordingly.

While some say I have some natural talent for management, I know my graduate education has helped me become a better manager. A good program helps one identify one's strengths and weaknesses—capitalize on the former and overcome the latter.

My career has been rewarding and challenging. Many experiences prepared me for my present position, but my deep interest in policies that affect health care and my work in local politics have been pivotal to my successes. I urge nurses to become active, particularly in local politics, and to seek positions on boards and commissions that deal with health. Prepare to spend time doing it. Intelligent positions on issues require study and thought. You will also need to develop the strength to handle conflict—and the ability to occasionally stand alone for a principle.[1]

THE NURSE-ENTREPRENEUR

Janet Epstein-Baden, RN, CNM, and her colleagues, Marion McCartney, RN, CNM, and Barbara Vaughey, RN, CNM, are pioneers in one of the relatively new frontiers of nursing—independent practice. The three certified nurse-midwives own and operate Maternity Center Associates, Chtd., in Bethesda, Maryland.

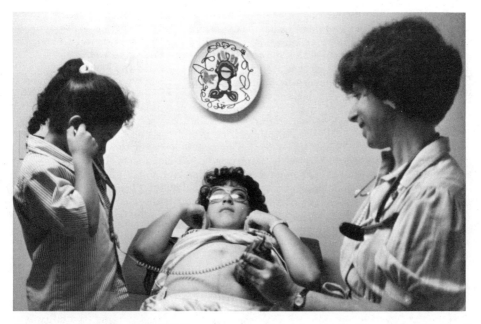

Janet Epstein-Baden, RN, CNM, performs a prenatal examination while the client's daughter observes.

The center has provided the services of nurse-midwives to women and their families in the Washington, D.C., metropolitan area since 1975. These services include prenatal care, birthing services at the center or at home, postpartum care, well gynecologic services, and family planning. In 1988 the center delivered 250 babies and cared for more than 1,000 women, including those seeking gynecologic, family planning, and obstetric services.

The center is housed in what was originally a four-bedroom family home. The waiting room, once the living room, bustles with activity. Mothers, fathers, and children all seem at home in this cozy atmosphere. The kitchen serves as the laboratory, and the place where routine prenatal blood pressures and weights can be taken and questioning can be done. Four examination rooms are on the first floor. The four labor and/or delivery rooms upstairs look like comfortable bedrooms—no equipment is visible.

How did it all begin? Epstein-Baden says:

> James Brew, MD, a Washington, D.C., physician who understood both the art and the science of medicine, had established a home birth service. While going against the grain of conventional obstetrical practice, his service became so popular, he was unable to handle it alone. He asked Marion and me to be "birthing assistants." Our job was to stay with his patients during the early stages of labor and to advise him when to come for the delivery. Our experience grew, and the arrangement worked so well, he urged us to become midwives, which we did.
>
> As I became more involved in midwifery, I realized that this was an area in which nurses could function independently. Nurse-midwives are concerned with healthy women and families. This was a nursing practice in which we would provide nursing services and hire physicians to perform medical services. We wouldn't need a doctor to function as a nurse. When we hung out our shingle in 1975, ours was one of the first certified nurse-midwifery practices in the country.
>
> We met resistance from the state Department of Health and Mental Hygiene, because the regulations governing midwifery did not fit our type of practice. So we worked with the state legislature to change the regulations to confine midwifery practice to those certified by the American College of Nurse Midwives.
>
> Another problem revolved around how we could be paid. At that time the part of the health code that regulated the practice of midwives prohibited their direct reimbursement by patients. Incorporation seemed to be a way to work around this problem. Fees for services could be paid to a "professional corporation," and the corporation in turn would pay nurses' salaries. However, to our amazement, when we applied, state officials told us that nurses were not on their list of "professionals," and therefore we could not establish this type of corporation.
>
> State Senator Rosalie Abrams, a registered nurse, intervened with the officials who had denied our request after I called her, asking for help. I opened our conversation by asking if she knew that nursing "is not a profession." Her response was "Oh, really?" Within 2 weeks we received notice that we could establish a "professional" corporation.
>
> Finally, we began working with Delegate Marilyn Goldwater for the passage of a bill that would mandate third-party reimbursement for nurse-midwives. During that time I became very comfortable testifying and lobbying in Annapolis. Under Marilyn's leadership and with the help of organized nursing, the bill was passed and signed.
>
> In addition to working out the legal problems involved in setting up our practice, we had to learn how to run a business. At the beginning Marion and I

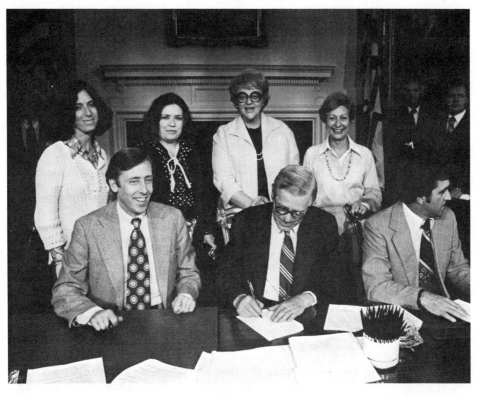

The bill mandating third-party reimbursement for nurse-midwives in Maryland is signed in June 1978. Back row, left to right: Janet Epstein, RN, CN; MNA lobbyist Lynelle King, RN; Maryland Senator Rosalie Abrams, RN; and Delegate Marilyn Goldwater, RN. Front row, left to right: Maryland Senate President Steny Hoyer (now a U.S. Congressman); Acting Governor Blair Lee III; and Speaker of the Maryland House of Delegates John Hanson Brisco.

invested $750 each. Then each of us bought $500 worth of stock in the corporation. We each loaned the corporation $250. What started on a shoestring is a business that now generates more than a half-million dollars a year. Becoming incorporated helped us become organized. From the beginning we needed the services of both a lawyer and an accountant.

We also needed the help of friendly physicians, pharmacists, and medical-equipment suppliers. At first we ordered medications, IV fluids, and equipment through these helpful supporters. Once we proved ourselves, we were able to operate independently. Dr. Brew—always supportive—was our medical backup until 1985.

There were myriads of other problems that had to be addressed. The center had to be licensed by the state and accredited by the National Association of Childbirth Centers, the organization which sets the standards for care and delivery. We meet the state and county codes regarding health care facilities. Laundry and autoclaving is done on the premises. Rooms are cleaned and cultures of the rooms and furniture taken weekly. We meet the community standards regarding screening lab tests. Our procedure book is 3 inches thick.

In 1985 and 1986 the withdrawal of malpractice insurance by midwives' leading provider created a major crisis nationwide. Most of the major national nursing organizations mounted a concerted lobbying effort in the U.S. Congress. Here in Maryland, Marilyn [Goldwater] and others worked with the insurance commissioner. The problem was resolved, but not without a devastating effect on our business. Fortunately, once we were insurable, our clients returned. But no matter how professional and careful we are, we are human. Malpractice insurance is an absolute necessity. We have a four-page informed-consent form, which spells out the risks of out-of-hospital births.

Our goal is to provide the service that we say we will provide in a safe manner. Ours is a business as well as a service. We must generate income, pay salaries, and do all of the other things that are required to be successful. No one considering embarking on such an entrepreneurial venture should consider it without being willing to spend a lot of time and energy on it.

We think consumerism is on our side. While we charge as much as obstetricians do for a delivery, the overall service does cost less than an obstetrician-managed hospital delivery, because there are no hospital expenses. But our selling point is that ours is a quality service. It appeals to a certain—usually well-informed—segment of the population. It is a challenge to work with our clients. Nurses are not threatened by their questions. We have something very special to offer. In health care and health maintenance we do a better job in caring for the family. In midwifery, nurses have opportunities to establish themselves as independent professionals who offer unique services.

For Epstein-Baden the years since she first thought of establishing a birthing center have been an odyssey toward self-actualization: "I conceived the idea, and it became a reality as a result of our ingenuity, blood, sweat, and tears. It has been successful. I love what I'm doing. I love nursing."[2]

MEN IN HOSPITAL STAFF NURSING

Identical twins George and Gregory Paul are civilian senior clinical nurses on different services at the Walter Reed Army Hospital in Washington, D.C. George works on the ear, nose, and throat (ENT) surgical service, and Gregory works in the emergency room.

The brothers were drawn to nursing when, as members of a Catholic religious order, they hoped to become medical missionaries in Tanzania. Nursing education was required, so they became licensed practical nurses. They were denied the opportunity to serve in East Africa when the Communist Chinese expelled all missionaries from the country. In time the two men left their order, worked as LPNs, and, shortly thereafter, entered the Prince George's Community College (Maryland) associate degree nursing program to become registered nurses.

William Fairchild, RN, MSN, was the first director of the college's nursing department and one of George's two early mentors. Ann Lombardi, a registered

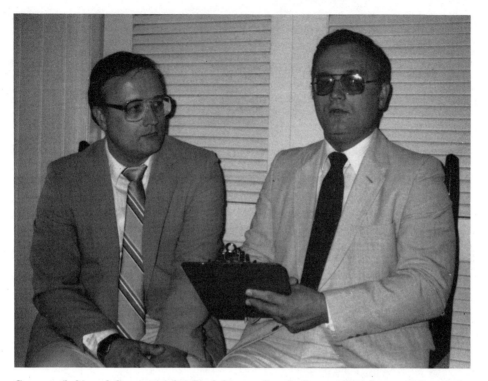

Gregory (left) and George (right) Paul discuss the challenges that face men in nursing.

nurse who served on the Prince George's County Council, was the second. Fairchild was a recognizably successful man in nursing, and Lombardi helped George find his way through the maze of politics in the county government.

Displaying a natural interest in and talent for organizational work, both men joined the MNA and have served as officers in their DNAs. Both men were active in the organization of collective bargaining at Prince George's General Hospital in Cheverly, Maryland. George has been his district's delegate to the ANA House of Delegates five times.

As part of a profession in which 97% of the members are women, George and Gregory Paul are role breakers. So what do these men see as the risks and the rewards for men in nursing? George says:

> Men can look at the profession as a guaranteed life career. Women tend to move in and out of the profession when they marry and have children. The problem for men is that salary compression of hospital staff nurses makes it almost impossible for a man with a family to stay at the bedside. While starting salaries are competitive with those of other professionals starting out, salaries of staff nurses usually do not increase proportionately with experience. In most cases a staff nurse has received his top salary after working 5 years in nursing. When there is no

opportunity for professional advancement, men either move, or apathy sets in. A man feels compelled to gravitate to administration, independent practice, such as anesthesiology, or industrial nursing.

Many men become successful administrators, and the proportion of men in nursing administration is disproportionately high, considering our numbers in the profession at large.

But for men who prefer direct patient care, we find that in hospitals, at the staff-nurse level, men are often assigned to the more technical areas, such as the intensive-care unit or the emergency room. Somehow, there is a perception that men are not sensitive, and if they were, they would be psychologists or social workers rather than nurses.

There are regional, cultural, and personal differences that affect the acceptance of men in bedside nursing. They center around such questions as, "Can a man touch another person and provide personal care for him or her?"

"Men learn very quickly in nursing school what they can say and can't," Gregory says. "Men believe they must be more professional, more efficient, and more circumscribed. Men are always under scrutiny. Men in hospital staff nursing are frequently lonely guys."

What then are the rewards that keep some men at patients' bedsides? Gregory says:

The rewards that keep women there. In some areas we can make special contributions. Some patients see men nurses as father figures. They feel support and strength with a man nurse. Many younger children feel very comfortable with men. The right man can have a calming and stabilizing effect on the staff. Whether rightly or wrongly, some people feel that a man can control.

Our experience in collective bargaining mobilized us for service to the community and nurses. We want nursing to be a profession worth staying in.

George says:

Since Prince George's is essentially a county hospital, as chairperson of our collective-bargaining unit, I went to Upper Marboro (our county seat) to try to promote the legitimacy of our cause. Ann Lombardi, as a nurse and a County Council member, was interested in health services and nursing. We attended work sessions of the council in an effort to understand the process and to ask for the council's support. We pushed for changes in salary schedules at the hospital that recognized differences in nurses' educations, work experience, and seniority. Members of the council listened to us, and while the results were inconclusive, salaries did go up.

In public forums we found that frequently when a man is in a delegation of nurses, the group is taken more seriously. Sometimes women are patronized. There is a perception that they are not strong enough to stand up, that their interest in an issue will be short-lived, or that ways can be found to work around their positions. So in this and other arenas we believe men in nursing have real contributions to make. Being men in an essentially women's profession is challenging, but we believe the rewards are worth the risks.[3]

A SENIOR VICE-PRESIDENT FOR NURSING AND PATIENT SERVICES IN A LARGE COMMUNITY HOSPITAL

Nursing administrators serve as the "bridge" between nursing and the other departments in a hospital. These nurses are sometimes caught between the needs of nursing staff and the often conflicting demands of hospital administration and medical staff. In these days of rapid change, top administrative positions in hospital nursing have become increasingly risky. However, in spite of the risks, some nurses find rewards in working out solutions to the difficult problems of maintaining quality patient care and the high morale of their staffs under trying conditions.

Rosemarie Liberatore is one of those persons who juggle the demands of their positions with apparent success. She looks on her job as challenging and rewarding. Her appointment as Senior Vice-President for Nursing and Patient Services at St. Joseph's Hospital in Baltimore in November 1988 expanded her responsibilities to include not only nursing but also housekeeping, laundry, dietetics, information desks, the switchboard, and the mail room. Liberatore believes that bringing these other departments under the same administration as nursing will integrate patient care services. She says:

> I have been in nursing administration since 1957 but have seen more change in the hospital arena of health care in the last 5 years than in all my previous experience. This new environment creates a real challenge. Under today's conditions our urgent need is to keep nurses in hospital nursing. My job is to give nurses the tools to do their jobs effectively, to make the environment in which they work

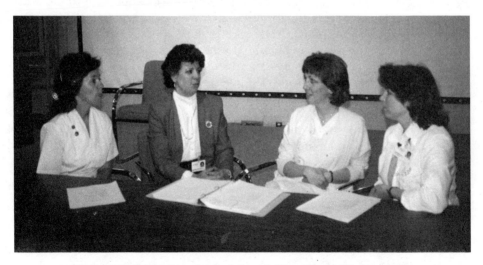

Rosemarie Liberatore (second from left) confers with her staff.

conducive to growth and professionalism, and to promote the delivery of excellent patient care. In my position I have opportunities to develop programs that improve both nursing practice and patient care, but I must often fight for the money to implement them.

At St. Joseph's we have instituted clinical ladders as a method of recognizing the staff nurse. By rewarding clinical excellence, we encourage her to stay at the bedside. Peer review committees evaluate the performance of nurses who want to move up, and recommend who shall be promoted.

We have also promoted unit-based practice committees, mostly run by staff nurses. They work in committees and help develop policies, standards, and protocols for their units. This gives nurses a great deal of control over their work environment.

The head nurse is a real nurse-manager. Her unit reflects her abilities and philosophy of patient care. Hers is one of nursing's most challenging and rewarding positions. In it she works with the staff, physicians, other departments, and patients' families. She is directly responsible for the quality of patient care on her unit. At St. Joseph's she may institute flexible staffing, allowing her nurses to work 8-hour shifts, but with the option to work 10- and 12-hour shifts in some cases. My job is to support her in every way I can.

In 1987 we instituted a flex pool for student nurses. We train them and then allow them to perform the nursing tasks they have learned. This is beneficial to us and also gives students valuable clinical experience. By the same token we are training volunteers to do some basic nursing tasks and have found that these volunteers are allowing nurses more time for real nursing.

As an administrator, you can never please everyone—and some things simply won't work. Some efforts are effective in one environment and not in another. When you see an approach won't work, you have to be willing to give it up. A manager needs to be very political. You need to know where the power—both formal and informal—lies. You have to work with people and know how to negotiate. Strategy dictates that sometimes you let others win, on the premise that you will win next time. A good support system within your department is a key ingredient of success.

Recognized for her management skills, Liberatore was appointed to the Maryland Board of Examiners of Nurses in 1982, on the recommendation of the MNA. She was appointed president of the board in June 1986. During her tenure the board has instituted a system of annual renewals for nurses' licenses, through which each nurse's renewal comes up during the month of her birthday. "This will give us current data about the availability and practice of registered nurses," Liberatore says. "It will enable us to plan more realistically in these days of nursing shortages."

The board has also streamlined its name, to become the Maryland Board of Nursing. Both of these changes required legislation, so board members worked with key legislators—especially nurse-legislators—to accomplish the changes. "I've found that the legislative process is the only way to achieve certain goals," Liberatore says.[4]

A COLLECTIVE-BARGAINING ORGANIZER

Nancy Pashby believes that an uncertain outcome is a necessary part of taking a risk. Pashby, who works two or three days a week in pediatrics and one day a week in home care, has been the chief organizer of the MNA's effort to organize collective bargaining at the Montgomery County Hospital where she works. Pashby is a risk taker.

In many states collective bargaining for nurses is relatively commonplace, but Maryland's legal processes make it unusually difficult to establish collective bargaining. As of December 1988 no collective-bargaining unit of nurses had been certified by an election process here. Given these obvious obstacles, why would an experienced hospital staff nurse make the effort to organize? Pashby says:

> On the basis of my 27 years in nursing I concluded that in some hospitals there is no self-determination for nurses without collective bargaining. I believe that nurses can be frustrated over a long period of time, but at some point they must take a stand. In our situation every single aspect of our work place is dictated to us—usually on the basis of financial considerations. In the year and a half since we started to organize, our nurses have always indicated that an improvement in nurse/patient ratios and the elimination of non-nursing functions—rather than salary increases—were their chief concerns. Our hospital management was so unresponsive to us that ultimately I could see no possibility for improvement in our work environment without collective bargaining. Both personally and professionally, I felt I had to try to organize a bargaining unit. I was determined to do so through our professional nursing organization, the Maryland Nurses' Association.

Organizing such a unit is no small task. First, the majority of the hospital's staff nurses must be persuaded to support collective bargaining. Pashby says:

> We have tried to talk with every nurse in the hospital personally. We hold meetings and publish a monthly newsletter. In it the case for collective bargaining is made, questions answered, administration arguments responded to, and membership and participation in MNA activities encouraged. Everyone writes, I edit, and members of the committee staple and distribute the newsletter throughout the hospital. The MNA district's newsletter is also widely circulated.
>
> We distributed and then collected authorization cards, which when signed indicate a nurse's interest in being represented by the organizing group. We learned the legalities, strategy, and politics involved in appeals to the National Labor Relations Board [NLRB], the final arbitrator in cases where hospital management and nurses cannot resolve their differences. We attend endless negotiating sessions with hospital management and hearings before the NLRB.

In May 1988 the group, under Pashby's leadership, organized demonstrations in front of the hospital demanding that the hospital allow nurses to vote on collective bargaining. Presenting her positions articulately and convincingly, Pashby became the nurses' chief spokesperson with the print and electronic media. Throughout the whole effort to organize, Pashby has been there—to listen, to persuade, to support, and to rally.

Beyond the problem of sustaining such an effort in a hospital at which some nurses become discouraged and move on, are there other risks beyond the possibility of not succeeding in establishing collective bargaining? Pashby says:

> While the law allows nurses to organize, jobs can be threatened. It is frequently difficult to prove that one is being disciplined. Personal attacks on the reputations of union organizers are not uncommon. I know that some people have

questioned my motives, suggested that I was publicity seeking and "bringing down the hospital." My relationships with my immediate supervisors have become more guarded—and this I regret.

Although the outcome of the effort to organize was uncertain at the time of the interview with Pashby, she still believes that her experience has been one of personal growth. She says:

My experience has proved to me that nurses must learn to work together for common goals and to be able to speak with one voice. In this and other areas nurses need to define goals and then adopt a team spirit that recognizes every person's contribution—no matter how large or how small. In my opinion, even in well-managed hospitals, administration—on principle—does not want to share power. A contract is an insurance policy for nurses. In difficult situations, rather than move, it is better to stay and try to improve your work environment—but it may require taking a stand.

When I look back, I will be happy that I did this. I have learned a lot about the democratic process, how to forge a consensus, and how to stay the course. In working with volunteers, I found it important not to give up on people, not to be critical of performance. If someone doesn't come through on one task, I try her again. Some

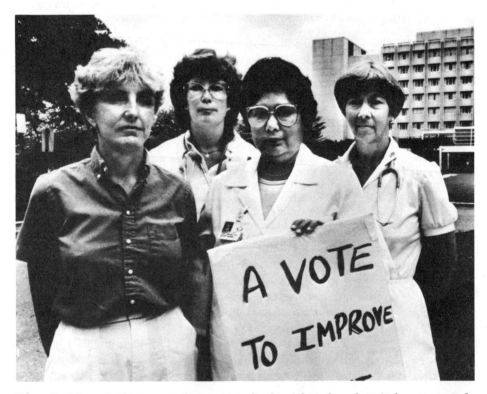

Nancy Pashby and other nurses demonstrate for the right to have hospital nurses vote for or against collective bargaining. (Photo by Dudley M. Brooks, *The Washington Post*.)

of the nurses who have become most valuable came into the effort late. Nurses are careful and cautious, and they wanted to be sure we were operating in a professional manner.

We've learned lots about the legal process and about negotiating. Successful negotiations require goodwill and a genuine interest in resolution of the problems on both sides. Leaders must stay flexible enough to find ways to accomplish goals. Give-and-take is part of the process. There are gray areas. We don't close doors.

Regardless of the outcome of our efforts I will remain active in my professional organization and a more active participant in the political process.[5]

A NURSE MOBILIZES OTHERS TO TAKE A STAND ON AN ISSUE

Amy Deutschendorf, a medical-surgical clinical specialist at Sinai Hospital of Baltimore, felt "enormous rage" when in June 1988 she read a newspaper account of the AMA's proposal in response to the nursing shortage. The AMA proposed the introduction of a new type of bedside care giver, the registered care technologist (RCT), who could be trained in 9 to 18 months to perform many nursing tasks. High school graduates from "low-income" groups were the pool from which RCTs were to be recruited. Deutschendorf says:

The AMA suggestion that registered nurses might choose to become RCTs was absolutely insulting.

I had never before become actively involved in an issue requiring political action, except when our children's school was scheduled for redistricting, but I was determined to do what I could to fight this proposal.

I started telephoning people I thought would have information, be interested in sharing it, or could be mobilized to fight the proposal. They included Maryland Nurses' Association Vice-President Judith Ryan (with whom I'd taught at the University of Maryland), the Maryland Board of Nursing, Maryland Senator Paula Hollinger (a registered nurse), and the delegate from my legislative district.

At Sinai the director and associate director of nursing allowed a group of nurses to organize to deal with the issue. We believed that rank-and-file nurses must be educated as to its importance, so we photocopied the proposal and distributed it widely. At nursing grand rounds I explained the issue's significance.

We formed a Resource Action Group. On July 18, 53 nurses from all of the clinical areas met to discuss how to acquire accurate and up-to-date information concerning the proposal, how to disseminate it to all nurses, and how to prevent the implementation of this proposal.

Local newspapers, radio and television stations were alerted to the furor the proposal was creating in the nursing community.

The day we held our first meeting, the *Baltimore Evening Sun* published a front-page story in which I was interviewed. (See pp. 146-147.) My own by-lined editorial appeared on the pages of that paper the next day. To my amazement it was headlined "Medical dumbness." (See box on pp. 148-149.) I wondered privately if my career was in jeopardy. Nevertheless, we submitted it (without the caption) to *Newsweek, Time, U.S. News [and World Report],* and *USA Today.* It was picked up by the wire services and used all over the country. We received responses to it from readers in New Hampshire, Pennsylvania, Washington, Indiana, Kentucky, and Utah.

Letters with packets of information went to Oprah Winfrey, Phil Donahue, Maryland Governor William Donald Schaefer, all Maryland legislators, hospitals

Nurses angered by AMA proposal
Plan would shift some duties to technicians
By Sue Miller
Evening Sun Staff

Nurses in Maryland and across the country, long frustrated by what they consider to be overwork, low salaries and little recognition, say they are outraged by an American Medical Association proposal.

The AMA plan would establish "registered care technicians," or RCTs, as a new category of hospital personnel to care for patients.

Angry nurses are mobilizing nationally to fight the proposal, which they say would lower the quality of patient care by replacing a diminishing pool of highly trained bedside nurses with technicians who have limited skills.

The proposal was endorsed, after much debate, by the AMA House of Delegates at its annual meeting in Chicago earlier this month.

The current estimated shortage of 300,000 bedside caregivers is expected to climb to 700,000 by 1991. Hoping to reverse the trend, the doctors approved three levels of RCTs, who would receive from two to 18 months' training at hospitals and community colleges.

The RCTs, both men and women, would earn as they learn before being hired. Their duties would range from bathing patients and taking blood pressures and pulses, to working in intensive care units. Their placement would depend on whether they were assistant, basic or advanced RCTs.

The doctors further recommended that the AMA Board of Trustees consider implementing pilot programs in parts of the country that are experiencing the greatest shortage of nurses who give bedside patient care.

Maryland and other East Coast states are included in that group, according to recent reports in national nursing journals.

When the word leaked out last December that the AMA was viewing the RCT concept as a solution to the shortage, the American Nurses Association and the National League for Nursing began setting up a series of summit meetings to work out strategies to combat the new category of hospital and nursing home health care workers.

The ANA, together with state nursing groups, has opposed the plan, stressing that the answer to the shortage is increased salaries and better working conditions for nurses, who for several years have been abandoning full-time hospital jobs for more lucrative positions in allied fields.

"Hospitals should start using more nurse's aides and licensed practical nurses, people they have begun to use less of in the last 10 years while relying on registered nurses to take over their duties," said Cathy Koeppen, an ANA communications specialist in Kansas City, Mo.

"The outrage is that the AMA proposal would replace bedside nurses with uneducated, unqualified persons and then it assumes that nurses would take responsibility for these persons," said Amy Deutschendorf, a clinical nurse specialist at Sinai Hospital and fac-

From the *Baltimore Evening Sun*, July 18, 1988. Used with permission.

Continued.

Nurses angered by AMA proposal—cont'd

ulty associate at the University of Maryland School of Nursing.

She contends that with RCTs the quality of care may erode and patients—who must be seriously ill to be admitted to hospitals under today's strict health care cost controls—may suffer.

An organization called the Liaison of Maryland Nursing Organizations met for the second time in two months Tuesday night in Baltimore to map the strategy Maryland will use to fight the new category of personnel.

"We just want to be included in discussions," said Kathi White, president of the Maryland Nurses Association.

"But the best solution to the problem . . . is to pay nurses what they are worth and get them back into the hospitals.

"The average nurse in this area makes somewhere between $26,000 and $28,000 a year and she has to work evenings and nights, weekends and holidays. Let's give them $20,000 more a year. Hospitals pay agency nurses these salaries, but they won't pay their own staffs."

The cry from nurses everywhere, according to Deutschendorf and White, is: Nursing assistants are needed to pass dietary trays, to provide escort service to tests, to empty trash that housecleaning misses, to run to the pharmacy for medication. But let nurses do nursing.

Dr. M. Roy Schwarz, the AMA's vice president for medical administration and education, said the doctors' proposal "may still be refined." He said the AMA Board of Trustees will not act on the proposal until it meets in October and after it receives an updated "status report."

That report will be drawn up following an Aug. 8 meeting in Chicago with national nurses organizations.

Schwarz, an educator who has spent 23 years in academia, said, "We have a problem—bedside patient care. No one is doing it. We have increasing complaints—in numbers and stridency—from physicians and patients.

"You've got to at least consider non-traditional solutions. Maybe this is not the best one. If someone has a better solution, the AMA would support it. Until that happens, we'll push for implementation."

Even if hospitals doubled nurses' salaries, Schwarz said, he doesn't think that would reverse the shortage.

"We no longer have a pool of young women interested in nursing to draw from and the opportunities for nurses have broadened too much," he said.

Dr. Michael J. Dobridge, president of the Medical and Chirurgical Faculty of Maryland, the state medical society, said Med-Chi has been besieged with letters from "all kinds of nursing people in Maryland, including legislators, like state Sen. Paula Hollinger, who are nurses" expressing concerns about what happened at the AMA conference July 1.

"We want to meet with the nurses and their representatives and discuss the problem in Maryland with them," he said. "We know that we have a progressively serious nursing bedside care problem. If the nursing organizations have an answer to that, then that's great with us."

and health agencies within the state, and to Marilyn Goldwater, who was a member of the Governor's Task Force on the Crisis in Nursing and was responsible for working with the public and private health care community to facilitate the implementation of the task force recommendations.

We notified television stations of a public hearing before the Maryland Board of Nursing regarding the RCT proposal. Two stations covered the hearing, which 300 nurses attended. I participated in a 2-hour radio talk show and was interviewed on one Baltimore television station in connection with stories on this issue. Our goal to bring the issue before the widest possible audience was being realized.

All nurses (including agency and float-pool nurses) were urged to write their legislators personally. For their convenience we posted lists of legislators' names and addresses in conspicuous places.

The board of the Maryland Nurses' Association met and asked me to help draft a flier alerting Maryland nurses to this threat to professional nursing practice—and outlining ways they could oppose it. The association assumed the expense of printing the flier and mailing it to every registered nurse in Maryland. The flier

Medical Dumbness

BY AMY DEUTSCHENDORF

Were you frightened when you were admitted to the hospital last month? Were you afraid that nursing shortages would affect your care? Did you receive the correct medicines? How long did you wait for pain medication? Did you think a private duty R.N. was the only one who could provide you with the level of care you needed? If you have ever had these concerns, you as the health care consumer may unknowingly be facing a more serious threat to your well-being.

The American Medical Association (in its infinite wisdom) earlier this month endorsed a proposal to deal with the current shortage of nurses. This proposal establishes a level of health care worker called the "Registered Care Technician" (RCT). This person will be a high school graduate with nine months of training and will perform bedside *nursing* functions such as the monitoring of vital signs, treatments (dressing changes, tracheotomy care) and the administration of medications. The RCT will be from "low-income" groups, will receive minimum wage and will function under the direction of physicians.

The side effect of this proposal will be more than the AMA bargained for. Rather than working with nursing to develop viable solutions for the nursing shortage, the AMA has further alienated current and potential nurses from entering a field which commands so little respect from physicians.

The proposal says that bedside care currently provided by nurses "requires relatively low levels of technology" and that an "R.N." may become an RCT if he/she "demonstrates the necessary bedside skills." This proposal verifies what all nurses have known for decades—physicians have no concept of what day-to-day bedside nursing involves, nor the level of training necessary to achieve it. This type of egocentric thinking has done more to unite nurses on a national level than any other issue.

The AMA says the reason there is a shortage of nurses is because hospital-based schools of nursing have been phased out in favor of baccalaureate degree nursing programs. In fact, the doctors ignore the real issue: Nurses have enormous responsibility,

From the *Baltimore Evening Sun*, July 19, 1988. Used with permission.

included an appeal for money to be used to fight the proposal. The response was gratifying. More than $5,000 came into the fund within a few short weeks.

At Sinai, bulletin boards in each nursing unit were designated as places to post information concerning the RCT proposal. The Resource Action Group paid $150 for 1,000 eye-catching buttons, which showed "RCT" with a "strike-out" [Fig. 9-1]. They were widely distributed to both doctors and nurses in the hospital. When given a button, each person was asked for a dollar donation. Money collected in excess of the cost of buying them was contributed to the MNA fund. MNA added its name but used the same design for anti-RCT buttons it distributed widely.

Nurses at Sinai actively lobbied physicians. We educated them regarding the undesirable effects on patient care, hospital and physician liability, and nursing practice that would result if the proposal were implemented. Packets of information were given to them, and their support in fighting the RCT proposal was actively solicited. Our director of nursing urged the Medical Executive Committee to pass a resolution opposing the RCT proposal.

On September 7, Senator Hollinger set up a meeting with representatives

---

Medical Dumbness—*cont'd*

deplorable working conditions and minuscule salaries with little opportunity for advancement.

In fact, the patient receiving care today on a general hospital floor was the intensive care patient five years ago. This patient requires a care giver who has extensive technical training and background in human physiology, pharmacology, social sciences and math. The nurse doesn't just disseminate medication and treatments—she evaluates their effectiveness and informs the physician of subtle changes in patient behavior that may indicate impending disaster. The attending physician may see his patient once a day; the nurse is the patients' last stand 24 hours a day in an environment that often can be hostile. The person who provides this care at the bedside must have a *higher* level of education and preparation—not a lower level.

Then there is the issue of cost and who will assume it. Many (if not a majority of) physicians are totally unaware of the impact of the AMA's proposal. The training and jurisdiction of the RCTs will fall on the physician and the hospital 24 hours a day. Nursing administrations cannot afford to assume liability for these poorly prepared health care providers, and bedside nurses should refuse to accept the responsibility of supervising RCTs. Therefore, the physicians' and hospitals' malpractice insurance premiums will most certainly increase. This cost naturally will be borne by the patient.

If the hospital environment was threatening before, you'd better be prepared to protect yourself before you enter the hospital. If you think staffing shortages affected your care previously, at least you had an advocate who protected you while you lay ill. If you're afraid that your primary health care provider is not meeting your needs, then perhaps you're better off at home. It is time for you, the consumer who ultimately pays for health care services, to take responsibility and refuse to allow physicians and hospital administrations to dictate the level of care you receive.

In the interim, don't get sick!

Amy Deutschendorf, R.N., is a clinical nurse specialist at Sinai Hospital.

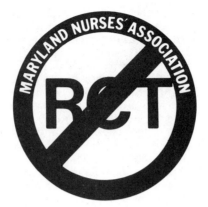

FIG. 9-1. An anti-RCT button distributed by the Maryland Nurses' Association. (Courtesy Maryland Nurses' Association.)

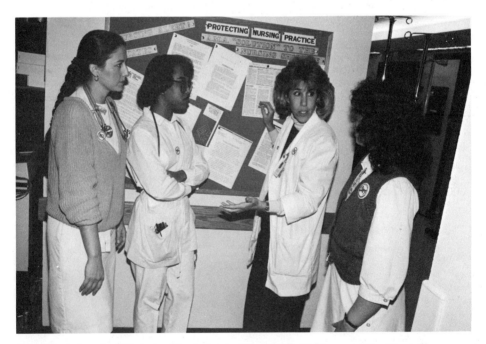

Amy Deutschendorf discusses the impact of the AMA's RCT proposal with staff nurses at Sinai Hospital, Baltimore.

from nursing practice and education, the Maryland Medical Association, the Maryland Hospital Association, and its Center for Nursing to discuss the RCT and alternate proposals for dealing with the nursing shortage.

Many credit Deutschendorf with being the key person in the mobilization of Maryland nurses' resistance to the RCT proposal. Deutschendorf believes that because of the all-out efforts of the Maryland nurses to combat this threat to nursing practice, the concept of RCTs will not be embraced by the medical community in Maryland. "The question now is: how can we help other states address this problem?" she says. "We are sharing our experiences with the ANA and other state associations."

What has Deutschendorf learned from the monumental undertaking? "You have a voice, and you can make a difference," she says. "First you must be knowledgeable about the subject. You must be able to sell your point of view. And you must involve your legislators, other policymakers, and groups of like-minded people."[6]

WHY RISK TAKERS AND ROLE BREAKERS ARE IMPORTANT

These, then, are the stories of seven nurses who have used their political skills, the media, and the political and legislative processes to achieve goals for professional nursing. Each in her or his way is a risk taker and a role breaker. Each has set goals that advance the profession as a whole, and each is typical of role models who can be found in every community. If you will look around you, you will find nurses you know who can provide the same kind of inspiration.

What makes some people strong, independent, and unafraid to take a stand in public? There are no simple answers to this question. It is apparent that some people set requirements for their own behavior that exceed what society expects of them. They see things from a different perspective and are able to mold their world, rather than be molded by it.

Common to several of our stories is the sophistication with which some nurses have learned to utilize the media. And all of them have found it useful to work with local politicians—especially nurses elected to public office. Nurses will probably always find it easier to work with nurses who hold public office than with other officeholders less well acquainted with the health care delivery system and our professional aspirations. We need nurses in elective office. Running for office is always a risk. Yet as nurses throughout the country become more experienced and knowledgeable in politics, more are throwing their hats into the ring. At this time, there is no way to keep track of the number of nurses who hold government offices. But as of January 1989 JoAnn Zimmerman, RN, was Lieutenant Governor of Iowa, Kathleen Connell, RN, was Secretary of State of Rhode Island, Barbara Hafer, RN, was Auditor General of Pennsylvania, and 45 nurses served in state legislatures.[7] Their names, addresses, and telephone numbers are listed in Appendix A. Nurses holding public office serve not only the electorate—they serve nursing. They deserve the support of not only our organizations but also the thousands of individual nurses. In the next chapter I will describe some of the realities, risks, requirements, and rewards of running for office.

Opportunities coexist with the challenges that face nursing today. We must have the foresight to capitalize on these opportunities. Now is the time to take control of our own destiny by meeting the challenges that face us.

We need articulate, knowledgeable leaders at every level of professional and political activity. However, not all of us are suited—whether by temperament or the circumstances of our lives—for the kind of path-breaking exhibited in the stories of the nurses told in this chapter. Even if we are not prepared to assume such leadership roles ourselves, each of us owes something to those who push out the borders that have traditionally confined nursing. We must support those among us who are innovative, creative, and willing to take educated risks in the belief that situations can be changed for the better. There is a job for each of us.

REFERENCES

1. Wilzack A: Personal communication, November 1988.
2. Epstein-Baden J: Personal communication, December 1988.
3. Paul George and Paul Gregory: Personal communication, personal interview, December 1988.
4. Liberatore R: Personal communication, December 1988.
5. Pashby N: Personal communication, December 1988.
6. Deutschendorf A: Personal communication, December 1988.
7. American Nurses' Association, Inc: Nurses statewide elected officials—nurse state legislators, Kansas City, Mo, January 1989.

Chapter 10

〃⁄ RUNNING FOR OFFICE

Running for public office is a lot like writing a book: the process requires 5% inspiration and 95% perspiration.

In a very real sense, your first political campaign begins the day you become involved in community affairs. Your work with your local PTA, school board, League of Women Voters, zoning commission, or political party will focus your interests, shape your approach to issues and problem solving, and help establish your credibility as a potential public official. The contacts you make and the friendships you form as you climb the community-service ladder will also prove invaluable when you finally take the plunge and decide to run for public office. Along the way you will also have the opportunity to earn a reputation as someone who gets things done, keeps your word, remains loyal to the party but recognizes the need to be nonpartisan on occasion, and rewards loyal supporters.

Although the road to public office, especially for women, has changed little since I entered politics 30 years ago, today's would-be politicians are much more deliberate in their pursuit of public office. While the genesis of my political career could be described as almost accidental, today most politically ambitious—and politically successful—women carefully plot their progress from school board to statehouse.

One factor in the increased interest in state and local races is the improved pay. Just before I entered the House of Delegates in 1974, Maryland state legislators earned $6,000 a year. By the time I left in 1986, their annual pay had increased more than threefold to $20,000.

Today people, particularly women, are starting earlier and aiming higher. Many of them are not willing to labor in the political vineyards as volunteers for years before they run for public office. And some may skip the school board and start with the state legislature. Regardless of the route you choose, you will need a solid base of community support to be successful. If you don't have this support, you will need a substantial amount of money. Preferably you should have both.

Lack of adequate campaign funding is a problem that has always plagued women candidates and probably will continue to do so for years to come. It has been difficult for them to raise money partly because they traditionally have not had the ties to the business community that their male counterparts have had. Only through many hours of unpaid community service have women been able to achieve the kind of visibility and credibility that only money could otherwise buy.

I have been asked many times how I got to be a state legislator. My experience is fairly typical of the experiences of many women of my generation who currently hold local, state, and federal office. Congresswoman Lynn Martin, one of the most powerful and visible women in Republican politics, is an outstanding example of the route that I followed. A former high school teacher of government, economics, and English, Representative Martin's political career began in 1972 with her election to the Winnebago County (Illinois) Board. After one term she was elected to the Illinois House of Representatives in 1976 and then to the State Senate in 1978. She has served in Congress since her election in 1980. Profiled by *Washington Woman* magazine as "the girl who's become one of the boys," Representative Martin became the first and only woman ever elected to the House Republican leadership when she was chosen Republican Vice-Chair for the Ninety-ninth and One-hundredth Congresses.

In 1959 I became active in the PTA at the public elementary school my children attended. The area in which we lived was growing rapidly, but the school system's growth was not keeping pace with the expanding school-age population.

The PTA Board, of which I was a member, supported the construction of another school in our area, thus beginning a carefully orchestrated campaign to obtain the funding. Proponents of a new school met with school board members, lobbied county and state officials, and mobilized the most important constituency of all—the parents whose children would benefit from the construction of a new school. It was in this first campaign that I learned a valuable political lesson: there is no special interest as powerful as self-interest. To avoid being misunderstood, I want to emphasize that I mean that statement in the most positive sense. Voters will back a candidate or an elected official if they feel that he or she has their best interests at heart. They also seem to have an uncanny ability to sense when their interests are not being served, especially at the local level.

My success in helping to secure funding for the new school encouraged me to become more involved in community affairs. I joined the League of Women Voters and became active in the local Democratic Party organization. Gradually I assumed more responsibilities in the Democratic Club I had joined. Our county's Democratic Central Committee asked me to take on a variety of tasks in several elections. While I passed out leaflets at shopping centers, organized candidate coffees, assisted at election forums, and directed volunteers, I was also learning valuable political skills.

I found politics fascinating and rewarding. Several candidates for whom I worked won election. As a result I asked for and received appointments to a county health board and a state higher-education board.

In 1974 an opportunity arose to run for the state legislature. Friends and fellow Democratic activists urged me to run. I was at a crossroads in my life. My children were grown and out of the house, and I was thinking about returning to school. I had to make what at the time was a difficult decision for me—should I take the chance and run for office? My husband solved the problem. "Run," he said, "and if you lose—but you won't—you can always go back to school." And so I took the plunge.

Being a candidate is very different from being a volunteer for a candidate. The candidate is always "on," constantly being scrutinized and assessed by diverse groups of potential supporters. In one respect an election campaign is a lot like an effort to enact legislation. In both situations your first job is to identify actual and potential supporters and opponents, as well as those who are undecided. Your next job is to convert the undecided, and your final job is to hold on to supporters and make sure they vote. This last step may seem simplistic, but remember that many candidates have lost close elections because they took their supporters for granted.

Once you decide to run for office, you must put together a campaign organization. The size and complexity of your operation will depend on the office you are seeking and the size and population of the district. However, there are features common to every campaign organization. Some are dictated by political practice; others may be mandated by state and local laws. Every campaign begins with a committee, and every committee has a chairperson and a treasurer. The committee chairperson may be a close personal friend, a professional colleague, the leader of a powerful constituent group that would benefit from your election, or a respected community leader. This person may restrict his or her role to administrative responsibilities and delegate issue development to others or may become a key political advisor who takes an active role in shaping your public persona.

It is helpful if your treasurer is a prominent businessperson or has close ties to the business community. The treasurer must fill out the required filing forms. Depending on state and local laws, the treasurer may have to file financial disclosure statements and prepare the candidate's financial report for the election. In many states these campaign forms are a matter of public record.

The finance chairperson's principal job is fundraising. There are many different fundraising techniques. In my first race, funds were raised by soliciting at coffees. Letters were sent to friends, relatives, and people I had worked with in the community. Some unsolicited contributions came from health care and education organizations. My finance chairperson and I made telephone calls to prominent Democratic contributors. Political parties can also be a source of funds.

Incumbency is probably the greatest asset in campaign fundraising. PACs contribute to incumbents without solicitation. Incumbents already have a base of contributors to solicit through letters and at events such as picnics, barbecues, dinners, and ice cream socials. For all these events you need a chairperson and volunteers to address invitations and attend to the many other arrangements. These arrangements include finding a location, hiring a caterer or

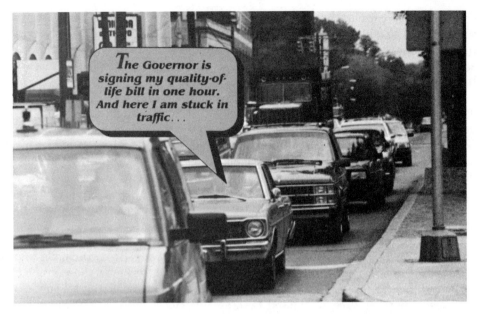

FIG. 10-1. Campaign literature addresses citizen concerns of traffic, the environment, and quality of life, August 1986.

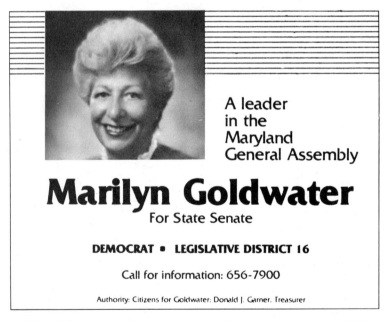

FIG. 10-2. Example of a newspaper advertisement, August 1986.

getting volunteers to do the cooking, deciding on decorations and entertainment, and making sure there are hosts and hostesses. Last but not least, you need a cleanup committee.

Ask your nursing colleagues, as I did, to host a dinner party for you. The dinner can be a simple buffet, with other nurses and their friends as guests. The hostess contributes the food, and the guests each pay $15 to $25. The candidate joins the group for dinner and concludes the evening with a few words about the campaign. I never found it easy to ask for money, and I am still uncomfortable. But realizing the need to have adequate financing for a campaign makes the chore more palatable. A former Speaker of the U.S. House of Representatives has made the point that people like to be asked—whether it's for money or their vote.

Although races for state and local offices are never as costly as those for Congress, the cost of running for these offices has risen sharply in recent years. My first campaign for the Maryland House of Delegates in 1974 cost $3,000. My last campaign (for the state Senate) cost $80,000 in 1986.

The increased costs of running for office are the result of several factors. With more women in the work force, there are fewer volunteers. Many experienced campaign workers want paid positions. The use—and cost—of printing and mailing campaign literature is up. Campaigns use more sophisticated polling techniques, more direct mail, and more radio and television advertisements. Computers have become an indispensable part of many campaigns. All these campaign aids are expensive.

Candidates need people to develop and track issues and to set a theme for the campaign, which is developed by addressing the concerns and problems of the voters. If you have been active in your community, you will know what these concerns and problems are. They could be the pace of growth and development, transportation (Fig. 10-1), the lack of affordable housing, the needs of elderly citizens, and, of course, for a nurse-candidate—health care. In my campaigns nurses wrote issue papers on all aspects of the health care delivery system and how it affects the profession and the public.

In urban areas polls are conducted by hired experts who analyze the area's voting patterns so that door-to-door campaigning, direct mail, and telephone banks can target voters receptive to your message as a candidate. Campaign materials must be prepared and distributed to reflect and reinforce your message to the voters.

One person must be responsible for coordinating press releases, contacting the media, and providing them with campaign news and dates of upcoming events. This person, the press coordinator, is usually involved in developing the paid political ads to be placed in commercial and organization newspapers (Fig. 10-2).

Someone is needed to direct volunteers—the lifeblood of campaigns. Whether a campaign has jobs as specialized as office manager and mailing-committee chairperson or one person manages both of these jobs as well as other responsibilities depends on the particular race, the candidate, and, of course, the amount of money available.

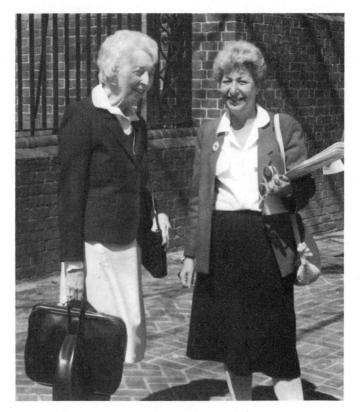

Delegate Goldwater campaigns door-to-door and meets a constituent along the way in October 1986.

Finally, a good scheduler, who acts as a "gatekeeper" for the candidate, is a key staff member in every campaign. He or she schedules your appearances and plans events so that your limited time is used efficiently and effectively. Arranging for and scheduling informal coffees, speaking engagements, shopping-center campaigning, and "door knocking" are all the scheduler's responsibility.

In fact a candidate's typical day might look like this:

6 AM	Wake up, eat breakfast, get dressed.
7 AM	Shake hands at commuter stations.
8 AM	Speak at a breakfast, meet with advisers to check campaign progress and schedule events.
10 AM	Campaign at suburban shopping centers.
Noon	Attend luncheon to speak and "work the crowd."
1:30 PM	Campaign door to door.
4 PM	Campaign at suburban shopping centers.
5:30 PM	Shake hands at commuter stations.
7 PM	Attend evening events—coffees, community meetings, fund-raisers.
10 PM	Check with campaign chairperson for following day's events.

In addition you will need to spend time on some days responding to question-naires and meeting with PACs and other special-interest groups that require a personal interview before deciding which candidates to endorse. As mentioned in Chapter 8, these endorsements are important because they bring workers and funds, as well as publicity, to your campaign.

If this schedule seems exhausting, it is. Many of my campaigns have been conducted at this hectic pace. A political candidacy is a lot like a roller-coaster ride: a lot of ups and downs punctuated by short periods of relative calm.

Campaigning is exhausting but also exhilarating. As a candidate you must always be on your "best behavior"—smiling, introducing yourself, and greeting people. When introducing myself—whether at a supermarket or a commuter station or in a neighborhood campaigning door to door—I often began like this:

> Hi, I'm Marilyn Goldwater. I'm running on the Democratic ticket for the House of Delegates. I'd like to leave my literature with you. There's a phone number on it so you can call me. Are there any issues of particular concern to you? Please call. I would appreciate your support.

As a candidate you learn not to stay too long at any one home. Cats, dogs, and children often become attached to you. You also learn just to greet people as they enter a shopping mall or supermarket but to give them your literature when they exit. Why? As shoppers enter, they are thinking about their agendas, not yours, and they are not in the mood to be waylaid. Literature given to them as they leave stands a better chance of going home with the shoppers and being read rather than being left in grocery carts.

The candidate coffee, a staple of most local and many state races, is a good example of how campaign machinery meshes together. In some ways it is a microcosm of the campaign.

In my campaigns, as in those of other candidates, volunteers arrive early at the host's home to take care of any last-minute details. They set up a table with campaign literature, pins, bumper stickers (happiness for any candidate is seeing his or her bumper sticker on a car, especially if the driver is unknown), plenty of name tags, and a sign-in list for later follow-up on the campaign's progress and possible volunteer recruitment. The host may have been recruited by my staff or perhaps by me on the basis of friendship, community standing, activism in past campaigns, or residence in a key precinct.

As guests arrive, volunteers make sure each one has a clearly written name tag so that I can address each guest by name. I begin my remarks by thanking the host and expressing my appreciation to the guests, follow with a brief (10 to 15 minute) statement on the issues, and conclude with a low-key pitch for contributions of time and money. After the event I send thank-you notes to the host and the guests. My staff members follow up later, trying to recruit additional volunteers from the guest list. These volunteers may in turn become hosts at future coffees.

Nurses were involved in every phase of my campaigns. I even developed a campaign brochure targeted at nurses (Fig. 10-3). Many nurses worked at the

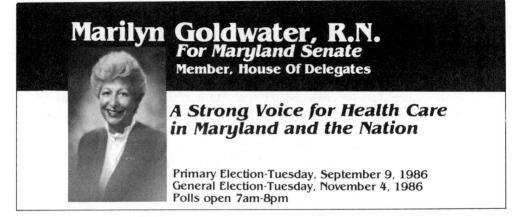

FIG. 10-3. Campaign brochure targeted to nurses.

polls on their way to or from work. In many cases they were particularly visible because they wore their uniforms. Many voters stopped to visit with them. They learned about me—and some learned a little about nursing.

Finally the big day arrives. At each polling place on election day there must be signs, as well as campaign workers to greet people, hand out sample ballots, and remind people to vote for their candidate. Staff members also serve as poll watchers and as drivers for people who might otherwise be unable to get to the polls. They staff telephone banks to make sure that people who have been identified in key precincts as friendly to their candidate and causes vote. As a candidate I always made the rounds of the polls and staff headquarters to thank workers personally. Then one or more volunteers at election headquarters would call in election results to me.

I always had a buffet supper at my home for my volunteers on election night so that we could await the results together. Then we would go on to a victory party at Democratic headquarters. Even when I lost my race for the state Senate, I went to the Democrats' victory party to congratulate the party's winners and thank those of my volunteers who had been unable to attend the supper.

A question that has been put to me frequently is "Why did you risk your House seat by deciding to run for the Senate against an incumbent, when you are keenly aware that 98% of incumbents are reelected?" I thought long and hard before making that decision and consulted with many people. These people and I believed that I had a chance to win, based on my record of effectiveness in the House. It has always been my position that more women should run for higher office, and I was willing to take the risk. It was a hard-fought campaign. Incumbency worked to my opponent's advantage, and I lost.

No one likes to lose a campaign, but the loss was not devastating for me. In my current position as Director of the Office of Federal Relations for the Maryland State Department of Health and Mental Hygiene, I am deeply involved in shaping health policy. I have learned a great deal about how the executive branch of government functions, and that has been a valuable experience. However, I do plan to run for office again in 1990.

So if you choose to run for elective office and then lose, make it a learning experience. Remember that success in politics involves luck and timing as well as hard work. Try again.

If you win, recall the last scene in the classic political movie, *The Candidate*. Robert Redford, in the lead role as the idealistic environmental lawyer-turned-packaged candidate, has just been rescued by his political consultant from an over-zealous group of supporters. The consultant sits the candidate down for what will probably be his last moment of peace and privacy for years to come and says, "Congratulations, Senator." Wide-eyed and slightly scared, he replies, "What do I do now?"

Read the next chapter and find out.

Chapter 11

⫻ YOU'RE AN INCUMBENT NOW: LEGISLATIVE LIFE

Once upon a time, a young, little-known state's attorney was elected to a U.S. Senate seat previously held by a formidable elder statesman who had become known as the "conscience of the Senate." When this fledgling senator showed up to claim his office, fresh from a hard-fought campaign and clad in his customary casual attire of an old sweatsuit and torn tennis shoes, the building guard challenged his credentials.

"I'm Senator _____," the young man said.

"The hell you are," the guard replied. The next day the senator's picture was at every guard station in the Capitol.

Today he chairs a major committee, is frequently quoted in the news, and no longer has any difficulty being recognized.

Such is the power of incumbency.

Now you have that power. The good faith and hard work of many people have made it possible for you to use your energy and intelligence to shape public policy, touch people's lives, and maybe even be part of the making of history.

So what do you do now?

First thank your supporters. Make calls, write notes, and take out newspaper ads thanking the people who worked in your campaign and the voters who elected you.

Next get organized. Incumbency has its responsibilities, as well as its rewards. The voters have transformed you overnight from private citizen to public servant. Show them that their good judgment was justified, and *buy a big calendar!* Accept and extend as many invitations to civic and professional association meetings as you can. If you can't attend an organization's meeting, offer to meet with an officer or representative over breakfast, lunch, coffee, or dinner. Invite members of the organization to stop by your office at the State Capitol or at City Hall.

Constituents need to know early on that you are accessible, and you need to know what is on their minds. They are an invaluable source of ideas, support, and political intelligence. If you want to be an effective legislator, you must first learn to become a skilled listener. And there is always the next election to think about. Like it or not, it is a political fact of life that your reelection campaign begins the day you take office.

Probably the most difficult adjustments I had to make as a state legislator related to time and privacy: I never seemed to have enough of either one. I had to get used to people calling me at all hours of the day or night and recognize that this communication was an important part of the job. I also had to become accustomed to feeling perpetually behind. There is just never enough time to do what you need or want to do.

Each state has its own system for orienting newly elected legislators, but in all states the new legislator needs to learn how the legislature functions. State legislatures share many common features.

In Maryland the period from the November election until the swearing-in ceremony on the first Wednesday in January is a hectic one. The county delegation meets to elect a chairperson and vice-chairperson. Veteran legislators brief newcomers on local bills, delegation meetings, and issues. Then there is a 2-day briefing session at the state Capitol. The freshmen are introduced to bill drafters, budget analysts, and returning legislators. They are also given a tour of the state campus and shown their offices.

Then new legislators are introduced to the nuts and bolts of legislative life: how to fill out expense vouchers, how to make arrangements for an apartment or hotel room during the session, and how and when they are paid.

Dinner with the governor is the highlight of these whirlwind 2 days. Watching the veterans' ease and self-assurance with the governor, you wonder if you'll ever become "one of the boys." Although women would like to believe otherwise, the corridors of power in many state legislatures are still largely male preserves. Fortunately the complexion of power is changing, albeit slowly: more women are holding leadership positions on key tax-writing and appropriations committees, where the real power lies. Women have also served as state governors and as speaker, majority leader, Senate president, and whip in state legislatures. The pattern is being repeated at the local level, where the number of women serving as mayors, city council presidents, and powerful council members is growing. Ironically many of these women have risen to positions of power because of their financial expertise. Houston Mayor Kathy Whitmire, an accountant, is an outstanding example. Vermont Governor Madeleine Kunin was the first woman to chair the Vermont House Appropriations Committee. She earned a reputation as a bright, effective legislator, partly by becoming expert in a somewhat arcane but important area for states in the 1970s: states' legislative appropriation of federal funds.

The parties caucus and elect their leaders, but it is not until the first day of the legislative session that the House and Senate elect their leaders. The Maryland House of Delegates is dominated by Democrats (141:17 in the House, 47:7 in the Senate), as are the legislatures of many mid-Atlantic and Southern states. Therefore, the House and Senate leaders also serve as the Democratic Caucus leaders. The Republicans also elect their caucus, House, and Senate leaders.

Selecting personal staff for legislators in Maryland is not difficult because limited funds allow you to hire only a part-time staff member. However, it is important that this person be compatible with you and know your district. I was fortunate to be able to hire someone who had been one of my volunteers. In addition, I always had a nursing student serve as an intern during the session. Legislators in other states have the ability to hire one or more full-time staff members. In large, populous states such as Michigan and New York, where the legislature is in session throughout the year and a legislator's job is virtually full time, staffs are larger. Legislative leaders and committee chairpersons may have professional as well as personal staffs.

States differ widely in their handling of committee assignments and practices regarding additional committees, but Maryland committee assignments

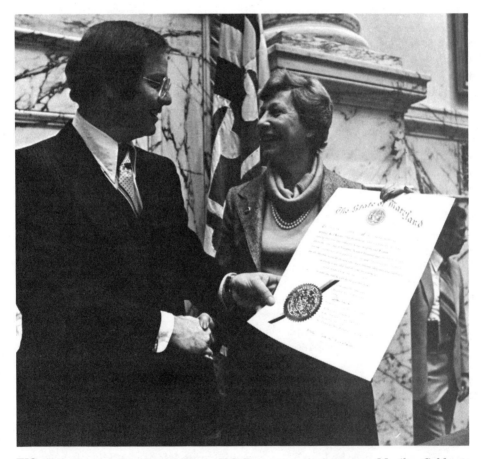

FIG. 11-1. Speaker Ben Cardin (now a U.S. Representative) presents Marilyn Goldwater with a certificate of membership in the Maryland House of Delegates in January 1979.

are made by the presiding officer in each chamber. Each chamber's leadership works hard at balancing the membership of each committee by party, geography, and sex. All members of the legislature serve on only one standing committee. However, a member can also get assigned to joint committees, special committees, or ad hoc committees, which all function during the 9 months between sessions.

One of the first things I did after my election to the House of Delegates was to write a letter to the Speaker, in which I designated my first, second, and third choice of committees. I was lucky enough to get my first choice—Appropriations. My colleague from my district and I were the first women to serve on the Appropriations Committee. Serving on the Appropriations Committee is a good way to learn about the substance and mechanics of the state budget. I was also on the subcommittee that reviewed the Department of Health and Mental Hygiene's budget. After my first term in office I asked for a change of assignment to the Environmental Matters Committee, since all health legislation went there.

Legislators spend a lot of time doing a variety of things before the first day of the session finally arrives. Words cannot adequately describe the emotions that washed over me during the swearing-in ceremony and the other rituals that take place throughout the first day of a new term (Fig. 11-1). Families, friends, and campaign workers all attended. After the ceremonies I hosted an open house in my office. That first day is even more special than election night.

Then it's down to work for the next 90 days or for whatever period your state legislature is in session. The Maryland House of Delegates meets for 90 days. Starting time for the House and Senate from Tuesday through Friday is 10 AM. On Mondays they meet at 8 PM so that people who work during the day can see legislators in action. The legislative session is an exciting time in Annapolis. The galleries and halls are overflowing with people, and during the evening session legislators have the opportunity to recognize publicly the groups that have come to visit.

During the session my typical day looked like this:

6:45 AM	Wake up, get dressed.
7:30 AM	Eat breakfast alone or with constituents or a statewide group.
9 AM	In my office, work on mail, make phone calls, check calendar, prepare to testify on a bill I am sponsoring.
10 AM	House session. Early in legislative session, spend no more than 1 hour per day in session. Later spend 3 or 4 hours in the morning in session, as well as some afternoons and evenings.
Noon	Eat lunch.
1 PM	Attend committee hearings.
6 PM	Back in office, check mail, sign letters, return phone calls.
7:30 PM	Attend receptions, dinners. Rarely spend time alone.
10 PM	Back in room, read. Could be 11 PM or later when there are evening sessions.

Things move quickly—and constantly. It's like being in a pressure cooker for 90 days.

I am frequently asked how I became conversant in the issues that were important to my constituents and the rest of the state and how I decided what legislation I would introduce or sponsor. These questions are related to a third question: when does a legislator merely represent constituents, and when does he or she educate and lead them?

To educate myself on key issues, I found it helpful to talk with veteran legislators, as well as leaders of different constituencies in the community. I formed a local advisory committee that included leaders of the PTA and of health, business, and citizens' associations and met with them regularly to discuss issues of mutual interest. I also held town meetings in my legislative district to be sure that I heard the views and concerns of my "ordinary," or unaffiliated, constituents. Regular meetings with party precinct officials were also essential to my continuing education.

Much to my surprise, the lobbyists and statewide organizations and associations that were fixtures during the session also proved to be valuable resources. As a candidate I'd had my doubts about these groups: their motives were always suspect. As a working legislator who was deluged daily with demands for my time and support, I grew to appreciate them as a resource.

With the constraints of having a 90-day legislative session and only one—part-time—staff member, it is virtually impossible for most legislators to know enough about all the issues to vote intelligently. This is where lobbyists, statewide organizations, and associations can be helpful. The good ones can boil down complex and not-so-complex issues into a cogent form, allowing you the luxury of thinking about an issue before you vote. How will this bill affect the state and my district? Where will we get the money to fund this program? Is this the most equitable way to raise funds? Is this the most cost-effective and efficient way to address the problem? What are the alternatives, and how much would they cost? These are just some of the questions a legislator struggles with in committee and before a vote. "Mental indigestion" is a chronic problem.

Less effective lobbyists give you reams of undigested, inaccurate, or incomplete information, leaving you no better off than you were before. As a result, their cause or organization is less likely to get a sympathetic hearing—or any hearing at all. Many good programs have died or never gotten off the ground simply because their representatives were ineffective.

Occasionally you meet a lobbyist or association representative who is downright dishonest in his or her zeal to promote a point of view. Over time you learn who is reliable and who isn't, and you also learn to trust your instincts. More experienced colleagues are often helpful as sounding boards and teachers.

Once I had acquired some basic education about the needs of my state and district—and I say basic because learning to understand such needs was a continuing process—I was in a position to address some of those needs. An idea for legislation doesn't strike you like a bolt of lightning. Usually it comes from a single constituent or a group that identifies a problem they believe can be solved by enacting a law.

The first bill I ever introduced required that the state government set aside 10% of its jobs for part-time employment, with prorated benefits. Much to my

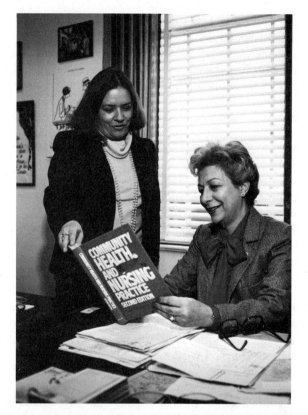

FIG. 11-2. Lynelle King, former associate director of the Maryland Nurses' Association, provides resource material for proposed legislation in January 1978.

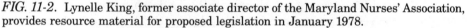

delight the bill passed and was signed into law. Another bill that I introduced and that became law required a picture on every driver's license. A third bill set aside a certain percentage of beds in institutions for the mentally retarded for respite care. When it passed, the law eventually allowed the families and other caretakers of mentally retarded individuals a break from their responsibilities in a way that ensures a safe, secure environment for retarded persons and a minimum of worry for their families and other caretakers.

Whenever I was planning to introduce legislation, I first talked with the executive agency that would be affected by the bill. If they liked the idea, they could be very helpful with budget and cost estimates and might testify at the committee hearing on the bill. Having the governor's support is also helpful. However, in politics people are free to disagree publicly with a policy, and the executive branch may also work hard to defeat your bill, regardless of its merits.

As a legislator I quickly learned that there are not just two sides to each issue. There are at least 12. Legislators have two responsibilities: to represent their constituents and to educate and lead. Handling the two is a delicate, diffi-cult balancing act. If you're doing your job right, you know the people in your district who are leaders on specific issues. You consult with them and listen to the witnesses at committee hearings. Legislative mail and telephone calls from the district also provide valuable input, as do lobbyists and association represen-tatives (Fig. 11-2).

Other good sources of input are the various groups, such as senior citizens, student nurses, or school administrators, that come to spend a day at the Capitol during the session. Their visits give you the opportunity to talk with them and hear their concerns.

But what if, after doing your homework, looking at all 12 sides of the issue, and touching base with your usual contacts, you still feel that you can't vote according to the best interests of your district?

It happens. What is good for the state, the county, or the city may not always be good for your district. Then it's time to put local, parochial interests aside and exercise another quality the voters saw in you: leadership. Later, regardless of the outcome of the vote in the legislature, you can use your vote as an opportunity to educate your constituents.

Fortunately there will be many times when you and your constituents have the same position on an issue being discussed in the legislature. And yes there will also be those times when nothing you do seems right, except to you. That's when you can console yourself with the thought that you must be a statesman. James Freeman Clarke said, "A politician thinks of the next election; a states-man, of the next generation."

If you stay in office long enough, you may also have an opportunity to serve in the legislative leadership. In Maryland the leadership is appointed by the presiding officer in each chamber. In most other states these positions are filled through election by the legislators of each party.

When I was Deputy Majority Whip in the Maryland legislature, I sat in on leadership meetings at which decisions were made on which issues the leader-ship would support and which ones it would oppose. The leadership also made decisions on procedures and on the daily nuts and bolts of legislative business. I was assigned about 17 delegates, and it was my job to check with them on their positions on bills when we were counting votes. Especially on a key vote legisla-tors should never, never assume that fellow legislators (1) will support them, (2) will oppose them, (3) will show up for the vote, (4) will remain undecided, or (5) won't change their mind at the last minute because of pressure from constitu-ents and other groups.

To help enforce the leadership's position, I would chat with each of my assigned members, tell them the leadership is supporting or opposing a particu-lar bill, and ask them if they would be willing to share their positions with me. I would always end with, "Hope the leadership can count on your help" and offer to provide any information that might influence their decisions in our favor. I would check with them constantly until the vote was taken to make sure that those who were with us stayed with us and to try to convince the undecided to vote with the leadership.

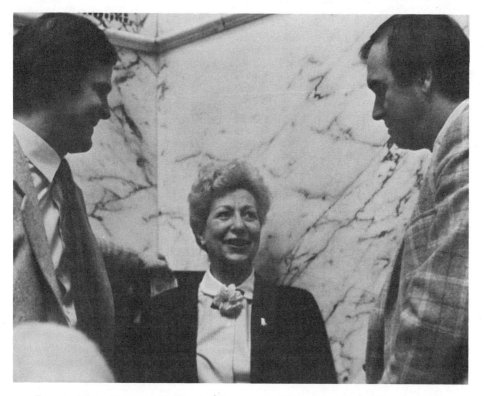

Deputy Majority Whip Goldwater discusses a bill on the House floor in 1985.

During the first year of my first term, freshman legislators formed the Legislative Study Group to work toward changes in the legislature, which had previously been the prerogative of the leadership. These changes ran the gamut from prohibition of smoking in the House chamber to reforms in our procedures through rule changes. The group also decided that we needed to raise funds to support the hiring of an executive director and to pay for office expenses; thus, the "Legislative Follies" was born. The group's talented members wrote, directed, and acted in this parody of legislative life, which is still an annual sell-out event.

The Women's Caucus also brought about much-needed reforms in the way state government operates and did much to change the traditional power structure of the legislature. We met not only to discuss issues but also to provide each other with moral support.

Throughout my 12 years as a member of the legislature, the attitudes of my male colleagues changed. The women in the legislature became a force to be reckoned with. First we addressed issues such as reform of rape laws, distribution of marital property in case of divorce, part-time employment with prorated benefits, job sharing, child care, child-support enforcement, and spouse abuse.

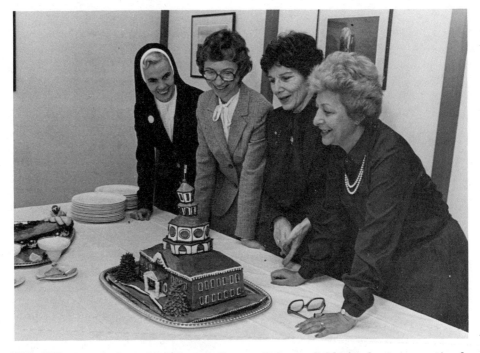

FIG. 11-3. As president of the Women's Caucus, Delegate Goldwater hosts a reception for women leaders in April 1981.

Later we looked at broader issues, such as how tax policy affects working women and families. We believed that although we called them "women's issues," they were really "people's issues," basic issues of economic self-determination, because what affects women affects all of society.

At first we couldn't get our male colleagues to cosponsor such bills. However, they eventually became more comfortable with the issues and very supportive of us; in some cases they even initiated ideas for bills.

Members of the Women's Caucus also became mentors to younger women by employing interns. The Caucus published its own newsletter and distributed it to all legislators, lobbyists, and women's groups. The group held an annual fund-raiser to support both activities. The growing success of the fund-raiser through the years has mirrored that of the Caucus. Few people showed up for the first fund-raiser, but by the time I left the legislature, it had become a huge success. The last Caucus fund-raiser I attended was also attended by our male colleagues in the legislature, male staff, and male lobbyists, as well as by women. Among our featured speakers were Lynda Bird Johnson Robb and Geraldine Ferraro. The governor gave a reception for caucus members and the speakers before the fund-raiser—that was when we knew we'd really arrived.

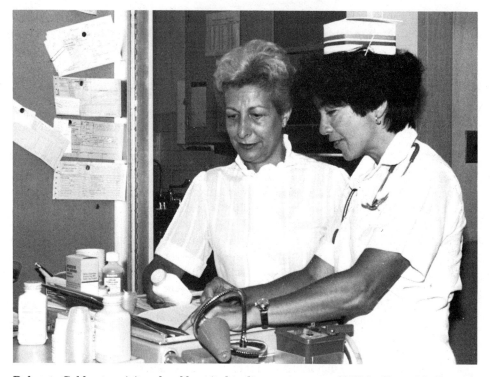

Delegate Goldwater visits a local hospital to discuss a proposed bill dealing with dispensing of medications.

I had the privilege of chairing the caucus for a year (Fig. 11-3). During that year we reached out to women's groups—business, professional, and volunteer—and, when appropriate, supported women's requests for appointments to boards, commissions, judgeships, and other key policymaking positions.

Another aspect of my job that gave me great pleasure was constituent services. One of the most rewarding and satisfying aspects of being a legislator is having the ability to cut through red tape for a constituent, to obtain hard-to-get information, solve a problem, or find a nursing home placement for an elderly person or a placement for a retarded child. I also enjoyed the regular, frequent direct contact that speaking to civic groups and holding town meetings in my district allowed. Answering mail and phone calls on pending legislation during the session not only kept me in touch with my constituents but also served as a useful check on my own political instincts.

Among the advantages of serving in the legislature in the decades since political reform are the sophisticated tools available to help legislators do their jobs more effectively. The "professionalization" of the nation's legislatures—the use of computers, the implementation of sophisticated techniques for budgeting and budget analysis, and the growth of and increased reliance upon professional staff—was accompanied by the creation of national organizations to serve state legislatures.

The Council of State Governments (CSG), with its headquarters in Lexington, Kentucky, four regional offices, and Federal Relations Office in Washington, D.C., serves both appointed and elected officials. CSG does research on state-related topics, formulates public policy on issues of concern to states, and publishes periodicals and reference books that provide up-to-date information on state government activities. CSG's studies and reports review areas as diverse as economic development, administration and management, health and welfare, and environment and natural resources. Their *Book of the States* is an indispensable guide to state demographics and is especially valuable when you want to sponsor legislation similar to that introduced in other states.

Another organization that is important to state legislators and one in which I was quite active during my legislative career is the National Conference of State Legislatures (NCSL). NCSL is the official representative of the nation's 7,500 state legislators and their staffs and is funded by the states out of their legislative budgets. The organization has three basic objectives: (1) to improve the quality and effectiveness of state legislatures, (2) to foster interstate cooperation and communication, and (3) to assure state legislatures a strong, cohesive voice in the federal system.

The organization accomplishes these objectives by publishing studies, reports, and periodicals (including a magazine, *State Legislatures*); holding well-attended workshops and annual meetings; bringing innovative state policies and initiatives to the attention of the media; and lobbying Congress and the executive branch. To help achieve this last objective, NCSL has 10 standing committees balanced by region and party that formulate policy on issues of concern to the states. I chaired the NCSL's Health and Human Resources Committee and served as a state spokesperson before Congress on issues such as Medicare reform and third-party reimbursement for nurses in advanced practice. I also chaired the Women's Caucus, which was not a policymaking body per se but served many of the same functions as our Maryland group.

I can't abandon the subject of legislative life without discussing a crucial issue—family support. Although my experience was made somewhat easier because our children were grown, it was still important that my husband share and support my efforts. Whether you have a spouse and children or just a spouse, they will need to understand—and tolerate—the fact that you will always be in the limelight, that your phone will be ringing constantly (frequently interrupting family meals), that people will approach you at restaurants and other public places, and that your schedule will always be hectic. In short they will have to learn to share you with your constituents.

Being a legislator means many things, but mostly it means putting together a mosaic, pulling all your efforts and resources together to work with the right person at the right time to solve everyday problems and to improve the quality of life for as many people as possible.

As a nurse I think I had a distinct advantage. Many of the skills I had developed in nursing were transferable: perception, sensitivity, problem analysis and solution, organizational ability, and the ability to work with people of different backgrounds and socioeconomic levels and people with problems.

Nurse-legislators have two other advantages that most legislative neophytes lack but which can come in handy for the sometimes frantic, often pressured legislative life: (1) nurses know how to be cool under pressure and tough under fire and (2) nurses are the infantry in the fight for human life and health. They are used to having a great deal of responsibility but getting little recognition or few material rewards for it.

Nurses are the ideal legislators: they come prepared for battle and poised to win, but they are also prepared to compromise and show compassion if they can advance the human agenda.

Chapter 12

POLITICAL PARTICIPATION FOR EVERY NURSE

In this book, we have walked together down the path of increasing political participation—from registering to vote to becoming an elected official. We have attempted to show through anecdote and description the highways and the byways of a fascinating odyssey that any nurse can take: personal involvement in the political process. Every nurse at some time in her or his life can and should step onto that road and go at least part of the distance with the nurses who have spearheaded the movement to use legislative and political clout in the pursuit of professional nursing and health-policy goals.

What we are advocating is an expanded role for nurses, both as citizens and as health professionals. Politics is pervasive in our daily lives—in our communities, our work places, and our professional associations. The more people participate, the more truly representational is our democracy. In contrast with a neighborhood swimming pool, in politics the more people who jump in, the cleaner it becomes.

The combined effects of what we do or don't do at every level in both the professional and public arenas affect the decision makers who shape health policy. Everything we do has an effect on the legislative, executive, and judicial branches of government and on the profession itself. Whether we like it or not— whether we choose to or not—we influence the political process. There are many actions we can take that can make a difference, but failure to act is also political. Failure to vote is a political act. Failure to speak up is a political act.

Health policy is increasingly being made by government—by elected and appointed officials who are not particularly knowledgeable about health care. They need to know that the health care system has many components and many groups of providers. Of these, nurses are by far the largest group numerically. We need to be keenly aware that health policy directly affects how we are educated, how and where we practice, and how we are reimbursed. If we are not involved in and knowledgeable about the legislative and political processes, if we do not take the time to share our views with those who make public policy, then we have no right to expect them to know our needs and the needs of our clients.

We believe that nursing and the issues that surround it as a profession—

174

such as actual and projected nursing shortages, health care–cost containment, accessibility of health care, scope of nursing practice, reimbursement, and advanced nursing practice—are major focuses of health care policy. They call for innovative strategies and coordinated efforts by the entire health care community to ensure a delivery system that meets people's needs today and tomorrow. They call for sensitivity and understanding of the work nurses do and the level of reward—economic and professional—they can expect for that work.

Nurses must take part in resolving these issues. We must set the standards for quality patient care. We must speak out on the ethical and moral issues affecting our clients. We must begin by expanding the focus on health policy in both undergraduate and graduate nursing programs. We must support the personal and professional development of every nurse. One way to do this is to encourage nurses to become active in their professional organizations.

Although there are nurses who as individuals have exerted significant influence and power both within and outside the profession, their full potential has not been realized because it has been personal rather than professional. They represent small groups of nurses but lack the support of a larger, unified group, which is necessary for the exercise of meaningful power.

Professional nursing organizations mobilize our collective power. Legislators perceive that the ANA and its constituent state associations address the broader issues in nursing and that the specialty groups speak to narrower ones. Therefore the cooperation of the ANA and SNAs with the other nursing organizations benefits us all.

Every nurse should be active in one or more nursing organizations. Participation in professional associations also provides personal rewards: the opportunity to form friendships with colleagues, have influence on issues in nursing practice, expand clinical knowledge, and hone organizational and political skills, which may be used in the broader political arena.

We encourage you to become involved in grass-roots politics in your own communities. That is the place most of us can make the most profound and immediate difference. Local governments deal with issues such as allocation of funds for public and school health. They also deal with planning and zoning issues, such as landfills, waste disposal, and building codes, which affect health, as do environmental issues, such as designated nonsmoking areas in public places. Initiatives that work in a local jurisdiction may set an example for other communities in the state or for the state as a whole. Legislation enacted in one state frequently becomes a model for legislation in other states—and sometimes for federal legislation.

We need, in local, state, and national political circles, nursing leaders with vision, people who can identify with other nurses and clearly articulate the issues of the profession and of health care in general.

We need nurses in public office. Whether they are elected or appointed, the high visibility of capable nurses in public office reflects well on the profession. Their position gives nurses access to people who are knowledgeable about nursing issues and who can directly affect health policy.

When Carolyne Davis became administrator of the Health Care Financing Administration in 1981, she became the nurse with the highest ranking federal appointment to that time. In this position she had remarkable influence on health policy. She believes that her tenure was beneficial not only to the public but also to nursing. Davis says:

> In working with legislators and testifying before them, I believe I was credible. Even those opposed to policies I supported found me knowledgeable. I felt I could translate complicated issues into language that legislators and the public could understand. I was respected as a person and as a nurse.
> I think my work with physicians' groups heightened their awareness that nurses are intelligent. We were working to resolve issues that directly affected them. They found me fair and cognizant of all their issues.[1]

You may remember that Davis, whom we met in Chapter 2, received her appointment not only on the basis of her experience and talents but also as a direct result of her participation in Republican politics in Michigan. Work in grass-roots politics within one's political party, then, is one way to gain the background and public exposure that are prerequisites for public office. Memberships on influential boards and commissions are another way to gain experience and recognition.

Achieving these positions of influence need not be a lonely road. Nursing organizations at every level can do much to promote these appointments. SNAs are frequently called upon to forward to the governor short lists of candidates for commissions, and DNAs have opportunities to recommend nurses for local boards and commissions. Every nursing organization should form a talent bank, in which the résumés of nurses who would be interested in such assignments are kept. Then, when opportunities present themselves, these organizations should be sure that recommendations are made.

Political or legislative internships provide yet another way to gain expertise in government. In Washington, D.C., some nurses have received excellent experience as interns in the ANA office and as White House or Robert Wood Johnson fellows.* Some legislators at both the federal and state levels hire nurses as staff experts on health care. These are opportunities to learn and influence that nurses with greater-than-average interest in health policy should explore.

The profession itself can do more to prepare nurses for leadership in the public arena. Barbara Curtis, RN, who has been a member of the ANA/PAC Board of Directors for most of the years since the PAC's establishment, believes we must do more to groom nurses for elective office. Curtis says:

> More experienced nurses must mentor potential nurse-candidates. We must say, "We will be there with you. We will help you build your network." Running for public office cannot be left to chance. It requires long-term planning.

---

*For more information write either White House Fellowships, 712 Jackson Place, N.W., Washington, DC 20503, or the Robert Wood Johnson Foundation, P.O. Box 2316, College Road, Princeton, NJ 08543-2316.

Early on, nurses interested in public office must realize that it is important to set up a home base where they live and that a party affiliation is significant. It is through precinct work that one can work oneself into the party. Would-be candidates should develop a card file filled with the names and telephone numbers of people they meet in local government. They should attend meetings of the county board to learn both the process and the players.[2]

Although helping nurses who are interested in public service to attain leadership positions is one strategy for increasing nursing's influence, there are opportunities for every nurse to make a difference through participation in the political process. Whether it be through studying the issues and articulating your position, participating in your professional association's legislative committee or PAC, lobbying for needed legislation, writing elected representatives, taking part in a campaign, or casting a thoughtful vote, every nurse's contribution is important.

Hundreds and thousands of nurses, through their participation in their PACs and in political campaigns, bring to the public arena their knowledge of what is happening at the bedside. Without them, health policy would not be tied to reality.

The voices of nurses, the profession's foot soldiers, must be heard. If we abdicate this responsibility, we have no right to expect policymakers to understand what the realities in the health care arena are.

We believe the future for nursing is bright if we resolve the issues of the present. The bottom line is that *we* must control our practice. If we don't, others will. Decisions made today will directly affect tomorrow's health care. We must increase mentorship and peer support if we are to have future leaders.

Every one of us must assume responsibility for the direction of both our profession and health care as a whole. We can influence health policy only if we are recognized as knowledgeable, respected as professional, and prepared to use our political power. Each of us has a personal responsibility for shaping a positive nursing image. We must learn to use the media to get our messages across to the public. We must know how to influence the decision makers and ensure that we have nurses in decision-making positions.

Today health care is the second-largest industry in the United States, employing more than 7 million people. More than 1.2 million of these people are nurses. Our influence must be felt. Effective political action is the prescription that will empower nursing to achieve greater influence.

A former Vice-President of the United States, Hubert H. Humphrey, said, "The moral test of government is how that government treats those in the dawn of life—its children; those in the shadows of life—the sick, the needy, and the handicapped; and those in the twilight of life—the elderly."

Our challenge is to use our influence to ensure that government meets this moral test.

What better legacy could we leave future generations than a unified profession that controls its own practice and exhibits leadership in the arenas in which health policy is made?

REFERENCES

1. Davis CK: Personal communication, November 1987.
2. Curtis B: Personal communication, November 1988.

APPENDIXES

APPENDIX A: NURSES WHO HOLD PUBLIC OFFICE
Nurses Who Hold Statewide Offices (1989)

Lieutenant Governor JoAnn Zimmerman,
RN
State Capitol
Des Moines, IA 50265
(515) 281-3421

Secretary of State Kathleen Connell, RN
State House
Room 217
Smith St
Providence, RI 02903
(401) 277-2357

Auditor General Barbara Hafer, RN
119 Courthouse
Pittsburgh, PA 15219
(412) 355-5301
(Republican)

State Legislators Who Are Nurses (1989)

Arizona
Representative Ruth Eskesen, RN
5771 N Placita Amanecer
Tucson, AZ 85718
(602) 299-3059
(Republican)

Arkansas
Representative Jim Lendall, RN
PO Box 55555
Little Rock, AR 72225
(501) 666-6100 (work)
(Independent)

4507 Kenyon
Little Rock, AR 72205
(501) 664-1398 (home)

California
Representative Tim Leslie, RN
1098 Melody Lane
Suite 101
Roosevelt, CA 95678
(916) 445-4445
(Republican)

Connecticut
Jacqueline M. Cocco, RN
93 Heppenstall Dr
Bridgeport, CT 06604
(Democrat)

Representative Norma Gyle, RN
6 Milltown Rd
New Fairfield, CT 06812
(Republican)

Hawaii
Representative Eloise Tungtalan, RN
State Capitol
Room 428
Honolulu, HI 96813
(808) 548-2211
(Democrat)

This list was provided by the American Nurses' Association, Inc.

Indiana
Senator Patricia L. Miller, RN
1041 S Muesing Rd
Indianapolis, IN 46239
(317) 894-7023
(Republican)

Senator Jean Leising, RN
State Capitol
Indianapolis, IN 46204
(317) 232-3140
(Republican)

Kansas
Senator Norma Daniels, RN
130 Miles Ave
Valley Center, KS 67147
(316) 755-0394 (home)
(Democrat)

Representative Jessie Branson, RN
800 Broadview Dr
Lawrence, KS 66044
(913) 843-7171 (home)
(Democrat)

Representative Joann Flower, RN
RR 2, PO Box 2
Oskaloosa, KS 66066
(Republican)

Representative Cindy Empson, RN
PO Box 848
Independence, KS 67301
(316) 331-5712 (home)
(Republican)

Maine
Representative Betty Harper, RN
RFD 1, PO Box 120
Lincoln, ME 04457
(301) 256-5024
(Republican)

Representative Susan Pines, RN
22 Long Rd
Limestone, ME 04750
(Republican)

Christina Burks, RN
RFD 3, PO Box 2470
Waterville, ME 04901
(207) 873-0923
(Democrat)

Maryland
Delegate Donna Felling, RN
4701 Vicky Rd
Baltimore, MD 21236
(301) 256-5024
(Democrat)

Senator Paula Hollinger, RN
3708 Lanamer Rd
Randallstown, MD 21133
(301) 841-3131
(Democrat)

Michigan
Representative Margaret O'Connor
Capitol Building
Room 220
Lansing, MI 48909
(517) 373-1033 (work)
(Republican)

4300 Saline Rd
Ann Arbor, MI 48104 (home)

Representative Nancy Crandall, RN
3981 Norton Hills Rd
Muskegon, MI 49441
(616) 780-2450
(Republican)

Minnesota
Representative Karen Clark, RN
407 State Office Building
St. Paul, MN 55155
(612) 296-0294
(Democrat)

2633 18th Avenue S
Minneapolis, MN 55407 (home)

Senator Patricia Pariseau, RN
25660 Biscayne Ave W
Farmington, MN 55024-9303
(612) 463-8496 (home)
(Democrat)

New Hampshire
Representative Ada L Mace, RN
13 Sirod Rd
Windham, NH 03087
(603) 434-5285
(Republican)

Representative Ann Torr, RN
1 Old Littleworth Rd
Dover, NH 03820
(603) 742-7607 (home)
(603) 742-5807 (work)
(Republican)

Representative Katherine Foster, RN
110 Arch St, #32
Keene, NH 03431
(603) 352-5772 (home)
(Democrat)

Representative Irene Pratt, RN
66 Clark Rd
Winchester, NH 03470
(603) 239-4597 (home)
(Democrat)

Representative Jeanette Barry, RN
51 West Elmwood Ave
Manchester, NH 03103
(603) 625-8174 (home)
(Republican)

Representative Cecelia Kane, RN
391 Colonial Dr
Portsmith, NH 03801
(603) 436-5100 (work)
(Democrat)

Representative Katherine Hoelzel, RN
15 Dudley Rd
Raymond, NH 03077
(603) 895-3872 (work)
(Republican)

Representative Alice Ziegra, RN
RFD 1, PO Box 165
Alton, NH 03809
(603) 875-2151 (home)
(603) 755-2202 (work)
(Republican)

Representative Elizabeth Moore, RN
Cochran Hill Rd
New Boston, NH 03070
(603) 487-3363 (home)
(Republican)

North Dakota
Representative Judy L DeMers, RN
1826 Lewis Blvd
Grand Forks, ND 58201
(701) 777-4221
(Democrat)

Representative Pat DeMers, RN
RR 1, PO Box 87
Dungenth, ND 58329
(701) 477-6232
(Democrat)

Ohio
Representative Joan Lawrence, RN
4567 Red Bank Rd
Galena, OH 43021
(614) 644-6711 (work)
(Republican)

Oregon
Senator Jeannett Hamby, RN
PO Box 519
Hillsboro, OR 97123
(503) 648-7185
(Republican)

South Dakota
Representative Mary Vanderlinde, RN
1201 N Minnesota
Sioux Falls, SD 57104
(605) 338-6501 (home)
(Democrat)

State Senator Jacquie Kelley, RN
(HCR 537-A-17)
Pierre, SD 57501
(605) 224-2684 (work)
(Democrat)

Texas
Representative Nancy McDonald, RN
Texas House
PO Box 2910
Austin, TX 78769
(512) 463-0622
(Democrat)

Senator Eddie Bernice Johnson, RN
Texas Senate
PO Box 12068
Capitol Station
Austin, TX 78711
(512) 463-0123
(Democrat)

Utah
Representative Paula Julander, RN
1467 Penrose Dr
Salt Lake City, UT 84103
(801) 363-0868
(Democrat)

Vermont
Representative Barbara C. Wood, RN
Woodland Rd
Bethel, VT 05032
(Republican)

Representative Mary Simpers, RN
166 Porter's Point Rd
Colchester, VT 05446
(Republican)

Washington
Representative Margarita Prentice, RN
6225 Langston Rd S
Seattle, WA 98178
(206) 772-6480 (home)
(Democrat)

West Virginia
Delegate Barbara Hatfield, RN
4220 Old Kanawha Country Club Rd
South Charleston, WV 25309
(304) 348-5536
(Democrat)

Wisconsin
Representative Judy Robson, RN
325 West State Capitol
Madison, WI 53702
(608) 266-9967
(Democrat)

Representative Walter Kunicki, RN
1550 S Fourth St
Milwaukee, WI 53204
(608) 266-9967
(Democrat)

APPENDIX B: POLITICAL SELF-ASSESSMENT TOOLS
Political Astuteness Inventory

Place a check mark next to those items for which the answer is yes. Then give yourself one point for each yes. After completing the inventory, compare your total score with the scoring criteria on the next page.

1. I am registered to vote.
2. I know where my voting precinct is located.
3. I voted in the last general election.
4. I voted in the last two elections.
5. I recognized the names of the majority of candidates on the ballot and was acquainted with the majority of issues in the last election.
6. I stay abreast of current health issues.
7. I belong to the state professional or student organization.
8. I participate (as a committee member, officer, etc.) in this organization.
9. I attended the most recent meeting of my district nurses' association.
10. I attended the last state or national convention held by my organization.
11. I am aware of at least two issues discussed and the stands taken at this convention.
12. I read literature published by my state nurses' association, a professional magazine, or other literature on a regular basis to stay abreast of current health issues.
13. I know the names of my senators in Washington, D.C.
14. I know the name of my representative in Washington, D.C.
15. I know the name of the state senator from my district.
16. I know the name of the representative from my district.
17. I am acquainted with the voting record of at least one of the above in relation to a specific health issue.
18. I am aware of the stand taken by at least one of the above in relation to a specific health issue.
19. I know whom to contact for information about health-related issues at the state or federal level.
20. I know whether or not my professional organization employs lobbyists at the state or federal level.
21. I know how to contact these lobbyists.
22. I contribute financially to my state and national professional organization's political action committee.
23. I give information about effectiveness of elected officials to assist the PACs' endorsement process.
24. I actively supported a senator or representative during the last election.
25. I have written to one of my state or national representatives in the last year regarding a health issue.
26. I am personally acquainted with a senator or representative or a member of his or her staff.

27. I serve as a resource person for one of my representatives or his or her staff.
28. I know the process by which a bill is introduced in my state legislature.
29. I know which senators or representatives are supportive of nursing.
30. I know which House and Senate committees usually deal with health-related issues.
31. I know the committees of which my representatives are members.
32. I know of at least two issues related to my profession that are currently under discussion.
33. I know of at least two health-related issues that are currently under discussion at the state or national level.
34. I am aware of the composition of the state board, which regulates the practice of my profession.
35. I know the process whereby one becomes a member of the state board, which regulates my profession.
36. I know what the letters DHHS mean.
37. I have at least a vague notion of the purpose of DHHS.
38. I am a member of a health board or advisory group to a health organization or agency.
39. I attend public hearings related to health issues.
40. I find myself more interested in political issues now than in the past.

SCORING: 0-9   Totally unaware politically
          10-19   Slightly more aware of the implications of politics on nursing
          20-29   Beginning political astuteness
          30-40   Politically astute, asset to nursing

Adapted from Clark MJ: Community nursing: health care for today and tomorrow, 1984, Reston Publishing.

MATCH WHAT YOU HAVE TO OFFER WITH WHAT'S NEEDED IN CAMPAIGN JOBS:

Examine the descriptive phrases within the four vertical columns, A through D, at the top of the page. Select the 10 phrases which best apply to you, choosing a minimum of two phrases from each column.

Place a check mark in the empty box below each phrase you select. Then, moving down the page, darken each circle below your 10 check marks.

ADD UP YOUR SCORE!

Counting from left to right, add up the number of darkened circles for each campaign job. Put the sum in the box marked "Total." Then rank the jobs from 1 to 20, beginning with the job with the highest total points. This ranking will give you a good idea of where you fit in a political campaign!

	"A" MOTIVATION					"B" PERSONALITY					"C" RESOURCES					"D" SKILLS					TOTAL	RANK
(Place check marks here)	Feel I should get involved	Want public recognition	Believe strongly in issues	Want to advance my career	Want to run for office	Like leadership role	Detail-oriented	Persuasive-articulate	Self-starter	Find routine work relaxing	Want to work part time	Can work full time or more	Can work election day	Want to work at home	Have access to car	Bookkeeping, typing, clerical	Planning, organizing programs	Hiring, supervising personnel	Writing, public relations	Telephone, personal sales		
Campaign manager																						
Headquarters coordinator																						
Finance chairman																						
Treasurer or assistant																						
Fund-raiser																						
Clerical support																						
Scheduler																						
Advancer or candidate aide																						
Press secretary																						
Speech writer, copywriter																						
Researcher																						
Coordinator of volunteers																						
Door-to-door canvasser																						
Candidate																						
Host, hostess																						
Phone-bank supervisor																						
Phoner																						
Election-day driver																						
Event organizer																						
Poll watcher-checker																						

APPENDIX C: ADDRESSES AND TELEPHONE NUMBERS OF STATE AND TERRITORIAL CAPITOLS

Alabama
State Capitol
Montgomery, AL 36130
(205) 261-2500

Alaska
State Capitol
Juneau, AK 99811
(907) 465-2111

Arizona
State Capitol
Phoenix, AZ 85007
(602) 255-4900

Arkansas
State Capitol
Little Rock, AR 72201
(501) 371-3000

California
State Capitol
10th at L St
Sacramento, CA 95814
(916) 322-9900

Colorado
State Capitol Building
200 E Colfax Ave
Denver, CO 80203
(313) 866-5000

Connecticut
State Capitol
210 Capitol Ave
Hartford, CT 06115
(203) 566-2211

Delaware
Legislative Hall
Dover, DE 19901
(302) 736-4000

Florida
State Capitol
(Senate: Capitol South Wing; House:
   Capitol North Wing)
Tallahassee, FL 32301
(904) 488-1234

Georgia
State Capitol
Capitol Square SW
Atlanta, GA 30334
(404) 656-2000

Hawaii
State Capitol Building
415 S Beretania
Honolulu, HI 96813
(808) 548-2211

Idaho
Idaho State House
Boise, ID 83720
(208) 334-2411

Illinois
State House
State Capitol Complex
Springfield, IL 62706
(217) 782-2000

Indiana
State House (or State Capitol)
200 W Washington
Indianapolis, IN 46204
(317) 232-3140

Iowa
State Capitol
E Tenth Grand Ave
Des Moines, IA 50319
(515) 281-5011

Kansas
State House
Topeka, KS 66612
(913) 296-0111

Kentucky
State Capitol
Frankfort, KY 40601
(502) 564-2500

Louisiana
State Capitol
900 Riverside NW
Baton Rouge, LA 70804
(504) 342-6600

From The Council of State Governments: The book of the states, 1988-89 ed, vol 27, Lexington, Ky, and Archer SE and Goehner PA: Nurses: a political force, Monterey, Calif, 1982, Wadsworth Health Sciences Division.

Maine
State House
Augusta, ME 04330
(205) 289-1110

Maryland
State House
State Circle
Annapolis, MD 21401
(301) 269-6200

Massachusetts
State House
Beacon Hill
Boston, MA 02133
(617) 727-2121

Michigan
State Capitol
Lansing, MI 48909
(517) 373-1837

Minnesota
State Capitol
Aurora Ave Park
St Paul, MN 55155
(612) 296-6013

Mississippi
New Capitol Senate Chambers or
New Capitol House Chambers
400 High
Jackson, MS 39201
(601) 359-1000

Missouri
State Capitol
Jefferson City, MO 65101
(314) 751-2151

Montana
State Capitol
State Capitol Station
Helena, MT 59620
(406) 333-2511

Nebraska
State Capitol
1445 K
Lincoln, NE 68509
(402) 471-2311

Nevada
State Capitol
Carson City, NV 89710
(702) 885-5000

New Hampshire
State House
Concord, NH 03301
(603) 271-1110

New Jersey
State House
Trenton, NJ 08625
(609) 292-2121

New Mexico
State Capitol
Santa Fe, NM 87503
(505) 827-4011

New York
State Capitol
Washington Ave
Albany, NY 12224
(518) 474-2121

North Carolina
State Legislative Building
Raleigh, NC 27611
(919) 733-1110

North Dakota
State Capitol
Bismarck, ND 58505
(701) 224-2000

Ohio
State House
Broad High St
Columbus, OH 43215
(614) 466-2000

Oklahoma
State Capitol
2302 Lincoln Blvd
Oklahoma City, OK 73105
(405) 521-2011

Oregon
State Capitol
Salem, OR 97310
(503) 378-3131

Pennsylvania
Main Capitol Building
Harrisburg, PA 17120
(717) 787-2121

Rhode Island
State House
82 Smith
Providence, RI 02903
(401) 277-2000

South Carolina
State House
Columbia, SC 29211
(803) 734-1000

South Dakota
State Capitol
Pierre, SD 57501
(605) 773-3011

Tennessee
State Capitol
Nashville, TN 37219
(615) 741-3011

Texas
Capitol
Austin, TX 78711
(512) 463-4630

Utah
State Capitol Building
Salt Lake City, UT 84114
(801) 538-3000

Vermont
State House
Montpelier, VT 05602
(802) 828-1110

Virginia
State Capitol
(Senate Addition or House Addition)
Capitol Square
Richmond, VA 23219
(804) 786-0000

Washington
Legislative Building
Olympia, WA 98504
(206) 753-5000

West Virginia
State Capitol
1800 Kanawha Blvd E
Charleston, WV 25305
(304) 348-3456

Wisconsin
State Capitol
Capitol Square
Madison, WI 53702
(608) 266-2211

Wyoming
State Capitol
Cheyenne, WY 82002
(307) 777-7011

American Samoa
Maota Fono
Pago Pago, American Samoa 96799
(684) 633-4116

District of Columbia
District Building
Washington, DC 20004
(202) 727-1000

Guam
Congress Building
Agana, GU 96910
(671) 472-8931

Puerto Rico
The Capitol
San Juan, PR 00904
(809) 721-6040

APPENDIX D: A RESOURCE FOR UNDERSTANDING LEGISLATIVE PROCEEDINGS
Explanation to Facilitate Reading of Legislative Bills

[Light face brackets] are used only in bills amending an existing law. They indicate that anything enclosed thereby appears in the existing law, but that it is proposed to omit it from the law as amended. The brackets and anything enclosed by them are carried along into the law if the bill is finally enacted.

Underscoring is used only in bills amending an existing law. It indicates that the underscored matter does not appear in the existing law but that it is proposed to insert it in the law as amended. The underscored matter will be carried into the law if the bill is finally enacted.

[**Dark**] face brackets are used only in bills that have been amended, either in committee or on the floor of either House. They indicate brackets inserted by such amendment and have the same effect as light face brackets.

~~Strike out type~~ is used only in bills that have been amended either in committee or on the floor of either House. It indicates that anything so printed appeared in a previous print of the bill but is to be deleted and will not appear in the text of the law if the bill is finally enacted.

CAPITAL LETTERS are used only in bills that have been amended, either in committee or on the floor of either House. They indicate that the matter in capital letters did not appear in the original print of the bill but was inserted into the bill by amendment in either House. The matter in capital letters will be carried into the law, if the bill is finally enacted, in ordinary print, unless it is also underscored, in which case it will be printed in italics.

~~Strike out type~~ and CAPITAL LETTERS indicate only the amendments made to the bill at the last previous state of passage. All prior ~~strike out amendments~~ are dropped entirely from the new print, and all insert amendments previously shown in CAPITAL LETTERS are reset in lowercase type. The one exception to this rule is that a House bill amended more than once in the Senate or a Senate bill amended more than once in the House will, on the second and subsequent printings, cumulate all amendments made in the latter house, so that all amendments in which concurrence by the house of origin is required will stand out.

The line immediately preceding the title of the bill shows the stage of passage at which the amendments appearing on that print were made. All preceding printer's numbers of each bill are shown in consecutive order in a line at the top of the first page of each bill.

From the Maryland General Assembly.

Joint Resolution

The example on the next page shows a third reading copy of a joint resolution that originated in the House. It has gone through the committee process and is in its final version.

Note the status lines at the top of the resolution. They tell you that it was introduced by Delegates Goldwater and Kopp, that it was read for the first time in the House chamber on February 8, 1980, and that it was assigned by the Speaker to the Appropriations Committee. After studying the resolution, the committee gave it a favorable report, with amendments. The House adopted the committee's report and amendments on March 26, 1980.

The resolution was then printed in its final version, as shown, with the amendments added to the text. The resolution was then placed on a third reading calendar and voted on for the final time by House members.

Resolutions that pass are sent to the other house for study. Resolutions that fail are dead.*

---

*From the *Student Legislative Handbook,* Maryland General Assembly, Annapolis, Md.

Status Paragraph House of Origin Resolution Number Type of Legislation

```
                    HOUSE JOINT RESOLUTION No. 102
01 3475

---------------------------------------------------------------
By: Delegates Goldwater and Kopp                              27
Introduced and read first time: February 8, 1980             28
Assigned to: Appropriations                                  31
                                                             32
---------------------------------------------------------------
Committee Report: Favorable with amendments                  33
House action: Adopted                                        34
Read second time: March 26, 1980                             35
                                                             36
---------------------------------------------------------------

            RESOLUTION NO.  _____                       39

            HOUSE JOINT RESOLUTION                           41

A House Joint Resolution concerning                          45

        Examination of Nonbudgeted Funds                     48

FOR the purpose of requesting the Department of Budget and   52
    Fiscal Planning to review all nonbudgeted fund accounts  53
    and justify them to the General Assembly.                54

                    Preamble                                 56

    WHEREAS, Significant sums of money are expended in        59
nonbudgeted fund accounts which do not appear in the State   60
budget; and                                                  61

    WHEREAS, The people of this State have a right to be      62
aware of the expenditures of State funds and the reason for  63
such expenditures; now, therefore, be it                     64

    RESOLVED BY THE GENERAL ASSEMBLY OF MARYLAND, That:       66

    1. The Secretary of the Department of Budget and         68
Fiscal Planning is requested to review every nonbudgeted     69
fund account on the records of the Comptroller that pertains 70
to any agency of the State.                                  71

    2. The Secretary shall report to the General Assembly,   72
by September December 1, 1980, every nonbudgeted fund        73
account, the fiscal activity of that account, and the        74
justification for that account not being included in the     75
annual State budget; and, be it further                      76

    RESOLVED, That copies of this Resolution be sent to the  77
Honorable Louis L. Goldstein, Comptroller of the Treasury;   78
and the Honorable Thomas W. Schmidt, Secretary of Budget and 79
Fiscal Planning.                                             80


---------------------------------------------------------------
EXPLANATION:
    Underlining indicates amendments to bill.
    Strike--out indicates matter stricken by amendment.
```

Third Reader House Joint Resolution.

First and Third Reader Senate Bills

Shown on the next two pages are copies of the same bill. A bill's first draft is called a First Reader Bill. A copy of it is assigned to a committee for study by the President of the Senate if the bill originates in the Senate or by the Speaker of the House if it is introduced in the House.

The final version of the same bill is shown on p. 194. Note the changes made by amendments in lines 51 and 52 and 75-81. This final version is called a third reader bill. All changes made to the bill that are adopted by the Senators are printed in the third reader version. The bill is then scheduled onto a third reading calendar for its final vote in the Senate (see p. 207 for a sample House calendar).

If passed, the bill is sent to the House. If it fails and is not successfully reconsidered, the bill is dead.

The second reading of a bill is done by means of a committee report (see sample on p. 205).

To tell the difference between a first and third reader bill, compare the following:
• A first reader bill has one status paragraph, and a third reader bill has two status paragraphs.
• Under the status paragraph of a first reader bill you will see "A Bill Entitled . . . ."
• Under the status paragraphs of a third reader bill you will see "Chapter . . . ."*

---

*From the *Student Legislative Handbook,* Maryland General Assembly, Annapolis, Md.

Status Paragraph House of Origin Bill Number Type of Legislation

```
                    S E N A T E   O F   M A R Y L A N D

01r1367                    No. 890


By:  Senator Rasmussen                                        27
Introduced and read first time:  February 11, 1980           28
Assigned to:  Judicial Proceedings                           31
                                                             32


                    A BILL ENTITLED                          35

AN ACT concerning                                            39

                Trespass —Agricultural Land                  42

FOR the purpose of providing that entry upon agricultural    46
    land is a misdemeanor under certain conditions; and      47
    providing certain penalties.                             48

BY adding to                                                 50

    Article 27—Crimes and Punishments                        52
    Section 579B                                             55
    Annotated Code of Maryland                               56
    (1976 Replacement Volume and 1979 Supplement)            57

    SECTION 1.  BE IT ENACTED BY THE GENERAL ASSEMBLY OF      60
MARYLAND, That section(s) of the Annotated Code of Maryland  61
be repealed, amended, or enacted to read as follows:         62

        Article 27  Crimes and Punishments                   64

579B.                                                        67

    A PERSON, WITHOUT WRITTEN PERMISSION FROM THE OWNER       70
OR AGENT OF THE OWNER, WHO ENTERS UPON ANOTHER'S LAND WHICH   71
IS DEVOTED TO ACTIVE AGRICULTURAL USE IS GUILTY OF A MIS-     72
DEMEANOR AND ON CONVICTION MAY BE FINED NOT MORE THAN $500.   73

    SECTION 2.  AND BE IT FURTHER ENACTED, That this Act      76
shall take effect July 1, 1980.
```

EXPLANATION: CAPITALS INDICATE MATTER ADDED TO EXISTING LAW.
  [Brackets] indicate matter deleted from existing law.
  Numerals at right identify computer lines of text.

First Reader Senate Bill.

Status Paragraphs   House of Origin   Bill Number   Type of Legislation

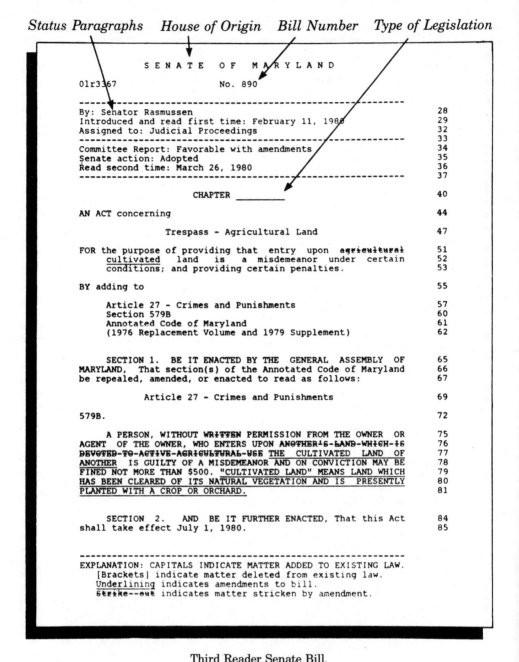

S E N A T E   O F   M A R Y L A N D

01r3367   No. 890

By: Senator Rasmussen   28
Introduced and read first time: February 11, 1980   29
Assigned to: Judicial Proceedings   32
                                                         33
Committee Report: Favorable with amendments   34
Senate action: Adopted   35
Read second time: March 26, 1980   36
                                                         37

CHAPTER _____   40

AN ACT concerning   44

Trespass - Agricultural Land   47

FOR the purpose of providing that entry upon ~~agricultural~~   51
    <u>cultivated</u> land is a misdemeanor under certain   52
    conditions; and providing certain penalties.   53

BY adding to   55

    Article 27 - Crimes and Punishments   57
    Section 579B   60
    Annotated Code of Maryland   61
    (1976 Replacement Volume and 1979 Supplement)   62

    SECTION 1. BE IT ENACTED BY THE GENERAL ASSEMBLY OF   65
MARYLAND, That section(s) of the Annotated Code of Maryland   66
be repealed, amended, or enacted to read as follows: 67

        Article 27 - Crimes and Punishments   69

579B.   72

    A PERSON, WITHOUT ~~WRITTEN~~ PERMISSION FROM THE OWNER   OR   75
AGENT   OF THE OWNER, WHO ENTERS UPON ~~ANOTHER'S-LAND-WHICH-IS~~   76
~~DEVOTED-TO-ACTIVE-AGRICULTURAL-USE~~ THE   CULTIVATED   LAND   OF   77
ANOTHER   IS GUILTY OF A MISDEMEANOR AND ON CONVICTION MAY BE   78
FINED NOT MORE THAN $500. "CULTIVATED LAND" MEANS LAND WHICH   79
<u>HAS BEEN CLEARED OF ITS NATURAL VEGETATION AND IS   PRESENTLY</u>   80
<u>PLANTED WITH A CROP OR ORCHARD.</u>   81

    SECTION 2.   AND BE IT FURTHER ENACTED, That this Act   84
shall take effect July 1, 1980.   85

EXPLANATION: CAPITALS INDICATE MATTER ADDED TO EXISTING LAW.
    [Brackets] indicate matter deleted from existing law.
    <u>Underlining</u> indicates amendments to bill.
    ~~Strike--out~~ indicates matter stricken by amendment.

Third Reader Senate Bill.

HOUSE BILL No. 586   2200-04810
(91r0458)

Introduced by Delegates Goldwater, Cumiskey, Hollinger, Rymer, Kernan, Bienen,   25
              Pesci, Harrison, and Douglass   26
                                                                                        27
           Read and Examined by Proofreader: 28
                                                                     29
                                                                     30
                                       Proofreader.   31
                                                                     32
                                                                     33
                                       Proofreader.   34
                                                                     35
Sealed with the Great Seal and presented to the Governor, for his approval this   36
                                                                     37
_____ day of _____ at _____   38
                                                                     39
o'clock, ____M.   40
                                                                     41
                                                                     42
                                        Speaker.   43
                                                                     44
               CHAPTER _____   45
                                                                     46
AN ACT concerning   47
                                                                     48
          Health Insurance - Benefits for Services   49
              of Nurse Practitioners   50
                                                                     51
FOR the purpose of requiring that after a certain date every health insurer, including   52
    any profit, nonprofit, and group and blanket health insurer, who proposes to issue   53
    a certain type of health insurance policy in Maryland shall ~~include~~ <u>offer the</u>   54
    <u>policyholder the option of purchasing</u> benefits for expenses arising from the care,   55
    treatment, or services rendered by a nurse practitioner; providing that the State   56
    medical assistance program (Medicaid) ~~shall~~ <u>may</u> pay for services rendered by a   57
    nurse practitioner; requiring the State Board of Examiners of Nurses to maintain   58
    certain lists; establishing a utilization Peer Review Committee to be appointed by   59
    the Board; and relating generally to health insurance policies for the services of   60
    nurse practitioners.   61
                                                                     62
BY adding to   63
                                                                     64
    Article 48A - Insurance Code   65

EXPLANATION: CAPITALS INDICATE MATTER ADDED TO EXISTING LAW.
  [Brackets] indicate matter deleted from existing law.
  <u>Underlining</u> indicates amendments to bill.
  ~~Strike out~~ indicates matter stricken by amendment.

2   HOUSE BILL No. 586

Section 354S, 470N, <u>and</u> 477T<s>, and 490A-3</s>   66
Annotated Code of Maryland   67
(1972 Replacement Volume and 1978 Supplement)   68
    69
BY repealing and reenacting, with amendments,   70
    71
Article 43 - Health   72
Section 42(a)(2)(ii), 294(a)(18), 295(f), and 301A   73
Annotated Code of Maryland   74
(1971 Replacement Volume and 1978 Supplement)   75
    76
    SECTION 1. BE IT ENACTED BY THE GENERAL ASSEMBLY OF MARYLAND,   77
That section(s) of the Annotated Code of Maryland be repealed, amended, or enacted to   78
read as follows: 79
    80
               Article 48A - Insurance Code   81
    82
354S.   83
    84
    (A) IN THIS SECTION <u>"CERTIFIED NURSE PRACTITIONER" MEANS A</u>   85
<u>LICENSED REGISTERED NURSE WHO HAS COMPLETED A NURSE</u>   86
<u>PRACTITIONER PROGRAM APPROVED BY THE MARYLAND STATE BOARD OF</u>   87
<u>EXAMINERS OF NURSES AND WHO HAS PASSED A BOARD APPROVED</u>   88
<u>EXAMINATION</u><s>, AND HAS BEEN CERTIFIED UNDER THE JOINT</s>   89
<s>REGULATIONS OF THE BOARD OF MEDICAL EXAMINERS AND THE BOARD OF</s>   90
<s>EXAMINERS OF NURSES</s>.   91
    92
    (B) AFTER JULY 1, 1980, EVERY NONPROFIT HEALTH INSURER WHO   93
PROPOSES TO ISSUE, RENEW, MODIFY, ALTER, AMEND, OR REISSUE A   94
HEALTH INSURANCE POLICY IN MARYLAND SHALL <s>INCLUDE</s> <u>OFFER THE</u>   95
<u>OPTION OF PROVIDING</u> BENEFITS FOR EXPENSES ARISING FROM CARE,   96
TREATMENT, OR SERVICES RENDERED BY A <u>CERTIFIED</u> NURSE   97
PRACTITIONER. <u>THE NONPROFIT HEALTH INSURER MAY LIMIT THE</u>   98
<u>COVERAGE OFFERED</u> <s>TO</s> <u>FOR THOSE SERVICES PROVIDED BY A NURSE</u>   99
<u>PRACTITIONER</u> <s>WHO WORKS</s> <u>WHILE WORKING DIRECTLY UNDER THE</u>   100
<u>SUPERVISION OF A PHYSICIAN.</u>   101
    102
    (C) AFTER JULY 1, 1980, A NONPROFIT HEALTH INSURER SHALL RENEW,   103
MODIFY, ALTER, AMEND, OR REISSUE ANY EXISTING HEALTH INSURANCE   104
POLICY TO <s>INCLUDE</s> <u>OFFER THE OPTION OF PROVIDING</u> BENEFITS FOR   105
EXPENSES ARISING FROM CARE, TREATMENT, OR SERVICES RENDERED BY   106
A CERTIFIED NURSE PRACTITIONER. <u>THE NONPROFIT HEALTH INSURER</u>   107
<u>MAY LIMIT THE COVERAGE OFFERED</u> <s>TO</s> <u>FOR THOSE SERVICES PROVIDED</u>   108
<u>BY A NURSE PRACTITIONER</u> <s>WHO WORKS</s> <u>WHILE WORKING DIRECTLY</u>   109
<u>UNDER THE SUPERVISION OF A PHYSICIAN.</u>   110

House Bill No. 586—*cont'd.*

Continued.

HOUSE BILL No. 586   3

(D) UTILIZATION OF NONPROFIT HEALTH INSURANCE BENEFITS BY A   111
CERTIFIED NURSE PRACTITIONER IS SUBJECT TO REVIEW BY A PEER   112
REVIEW COMMITTEE APPOINTED BY THE STATE BOARD OF EXAMINERS OF   113
NURSES IN ACCORDANCE WITH THE JOINT REGULATIONS OF THE BOARD OF   114
MEDICAL EXAMINERS AND THE BOARD OF EXAMINERS OF NURSES.   115
                                                                   116
(E) NOTWITHSTANDING ANY PROVISION OF A GROUP OR INDIVIDUAL   117
POLICY OR CONTRACT, OR ANY CERTIFICATE ISSUED THEREUNDER, OF   118
HEALTH, SICKNESS, ACCIDENT, OR DISABILITY INSURANCE, DELIVERED   119
WITHIN THE STATE, OR ISSUED TO A GROUP WHICH IS INCORPORATED OR   120
HAS A MAIN OFFICE LOCATED IN THE STATE, OR COVERING PERSONS WHO   121
RESIDE OR WORK WITHIN THE STATE, WHENEVER SUCH POLICY, CONTRACT   122
OR CERTIFICATE PROVIDES FOR REIMBURSEMENT FOR ANY SERVICE   123
WHICH IS WITHIN THE LAWFUL SCOPE OF PRACTICE OF A NURSE   124
PRACTITIONER, THE INSURED, OR ANY OTHER PERSON COVERED BY THE   125
POLICY, CONTRACT, OR CERTIFICATE, SHALL BE ENTITLED TO   126
REIMBURSEMENT FOR SUCH SERVICE, WHETHER THE SERVICE IS   127
PERFORMED BY A DOCTOR OF MEDICINE OR A NURSE PRACTITIONER. THE   128
PROVISIONS OF THIS SECTION SHALL APPLY TO ALL SUCH POLICIES,   129
CONTRACTS, OR CERTIFICATES ISSUED, RENEWED, MODIFIED, ALTERED,   130
AMENDED, OR REISSUED ON OR AFTER JULY 1, 1980.   131
                                                                   132
470N.   133
                                                                   134
(A) IN THIS SECTION "CERTIFIED NURSE PRACTITIONER" MEANS A   135
LICENSED REGISTERED NURSE WHO HAS COMPLETED A NURSE   136
PRACTITIONER PROGRAM APPROVED BY THE MARYLAND STATE BOARD OF   137
EXAMINERS OF NURSES AND WHO HAS PASSED A BOARD APPROVED   138
EXAMINATION, AND HAS BEEN CERTIFIED UNDER THE JOINT   139
REGULATIONS OF THE BOARD OF MEDICAL EXAMINERS AND THE BOARD OF   140
EXAMINERS OF NURSES.   141
                                                                   142
(B) AFTER JULY 1, 1980, EVERY HEALTH INSURER WHO PROPOSES TO   143
ISSUE, RENEW, MODIFY, ALTER, AMEND, OR REISSUE ANY HEALTH   144
INSURANCE POLICY IN MARYLAND THAT IS WRITTEN ON AN EXPENSE   145
INCURRED BASIS SHALL INCLUDE OFFER THE OPTION OF PROVIDING   146
BENEFITS FOR EXPENSES ARISING FROM CARE, TREATMENT, OR SERVICES   147
RENDERED BY A CERTIFIED NURSE PRACTITIONER. THE HEALTH INSURER   148
MAY LIMIT THE COVERAGE OFFERED TO FOR THOSE SERVICES PROVIDED   149
BY A NURSE PRACTITIONER WHO WORKS WHILE WORKING DIRECTLY   150
UNDER THE SUPERVISION OF A PHYSICIAN.   151

House Bill No. 586—*cont'd.*

Continued.

4   HOUSE BILL No. 586

   (C) AFTER JULY 1, 1980, A HEALTH INSURER SHALL RENEW, MODIFY, 152
ALTER, AMEND, OR REISSUE ANY EXISTING HEALTH INSURANCE POLICY 153
THAT IS WRITTEN ON AN EXPENSE INCURRED BASIS TO ~~INCLUDE~~ OFFER 154
THE OPTION OF PROVIDING BENEFITS FOR EXPENSES ARISING FROM CARE, 155
TREATMENT, OR SERVICES RENDERED BY A CERTIFIED NURSE 156
PRACTITIONER. THE HEALTH INSURER MAY LIMIT THE COVERAGE 157
OFFERED ~~TO~~ FOR THOSE SERVICES PROVIDED BY A NURSE PRACTITIONER 158
~~WHO WORKS~~ WHILE WORKING DIRECTLY UNDER THE SUPERVISION OF A 159
PHYSICIAN. 160
 161

   (D) UTILIZATION OF HEALTH INSURANCE BENEFITS BY A CERTIFIED 162
NURSE PRACTITIONER IS SUBJECT TO REVIEW BY A PEER REVIEW 163
COMMITTEE APPOINTED BY THE STATE BOARD OF EXAMINERS OF NURSES 164
~~IN ACCORDANCE WITH THE JOINT REGULATIONS OF THE BOARD OF~~ 165
~~MEDICAL EXAMINERS AND THE BOARD OF EXAMINERS OF NURSES~~. 166
 167

   ~~(E) NOTWITHSTANDING ANY PROVISION OF A GROUP OR INDIVIDUAL~~ 168
~~POLICY OR CONTRACT, OR ANY CERTIFICATE ISSUED THEREUNDER, OF~~ 169
~~HEALTH, SICKNESS, ACCIDENT, OR DISABILITY INSURANCE THAT IS~~ 170
~~WRITTEN ON AN EXPENSE INCURRED BASIS, DELIVERED WITHIN THE~~ 171
~~STATE, OR ISSUED TO A GROUP WHICH IS INCORPORATED OR HAS A MAIN~~ 172
~~OFFICE LOCATED IN THE STATE, OR COVERING PERSONS WHO RESIDE OR~~ 173
~~WORK WITHIN THE STATE, WHENEVER SUCH POLICY, CONTRACT, OR~~ 174
~~CERTIFICATE PROVIDES FOR REIMBURSEMENT FOR ANY SERVICE WHICH~~ 175
~~IS WITHIN THE LAWFUL SCOPE OF PRACTICE OF A NURSE PRACTITIONER,~~ 176
~~THE INSURED, OR ANY OTHER PERSON COVERED BY THE POLICY,~~ 177
~~CONTRACT, OR CERTIFICATE, SHALL BE ENTITLED TO REIMBURSEMENT~~ 178
~~FOR SUCH SERVICE, WHETHER THE SERVICE IS PERFORMED BY A DOCTOR~~ 179
~~OF MEDICINE OR A NURSE MIDWIFE. THE PROVISIONS OF THIS SECTION~~ 180
~~SHALL APPLY TO ALL SUCH POLICIES, CONTRACTS, OR CERTIFICATES~~ 181
~~ISSUED, RENEWED, MODIFIED, ALTERED, AMENDED, OR REISSUED ON OR~~ 182
~~AFTER JULY 1, 1980.~~ 183
 184

477T. 185
 186

   (A) IN THIS SECTION "CERTIFIED NURSE PRACTITIONER" MEANS A 187
LICENSED REGISTERED NURSE WHO HAS COMPLETED A NURSE 188
PRACTITIONER PROGRAM APPROVED BY THE MARYLAND STATE BOARD OF 189
EXAMINERS OF NURSES AND WHO HAS PASSED A BOARD APPROVED 190
EXAMINATION~~, AND HAS BEEN CERTIFIED UNDER THE JOINT~~ 191
~~REGULATIONS OF THE BOARD OF MEDICAL EXAMINERS AND THE BOARD OF~~ 192
~~EXAMINERS OF NURSES~~. 193

Continued.

HOUSE BILL No. 586   5

(B)   AFTER JULY 1, 1980, EVERY GROUP OR BLANKET HEALTH INSURER   194
WHO PROPOSES TO ISSUE, RENEW, MODIFY, ALTER, AMEND, OR REISSUE   195
ANY HEALTH INSURANCE POLICY IN MARYLAND THAT IS WRITTEN ON AN   196
EXPENSE INCURRED BASIS SHALL ~~INCLUDE~~ OFFER THE OPTION OF   197
PROVIDING BENEFITS FOR EXPENSES ARISING FROM CARE, TREATMENT,   198
OR SERVICES RENDERED BY A CERTIFIED NURSE PRACTITIONER. THE   199
GROUP OR BLANKET HEALTH INSURER MAY LIMIT THE COVERAGE   200
OFFERED ~~TO~~ FOR THOSE SERVICES PROVIDED BY A NURSE PRACTITIONER   201
~~WHO WORKS~~ WHILE WORKING DIRECTLY UNDER THE SUPERVISION OF A   202
PHYSICIAN.   203
                                                                        204
(C)   AFTER JULY 1, 1980, A GROUP OR BLANKET HEALTH INSURER   205
SHALL RENEW, MODIFY, ALTER, AMEND, OR REISSUE ANY EXISTING   206
HEALTH INSURANCE POLICY THAT IS WRITTEN ON AN EXPENSE INCURRED   207
BASIS TO ~~INCLUDE~~ OFFER THE OPTION OF PROVIDING BENEFITS FOR   208
EXPENSES ARISING FROM CARE, TREATMENT, OR SERVICES RENDERED BY   209
A CERTIFIED NURSE PRACTITIONER. THE GROUP OR BLANKET HEALTH   210
INSURER MAY LIMIT THE COVERAGE OFFERED ~~TO~~ FOR THOSE SERVICES   211
PROVIDED BY A NURSE PRACTITIONER ~~WHO WORKS~~ WHILE WORKING   212
DIRECTLY UNDER THE SUPERVISION OF A PHYSICIAN.   213
                                                                        214
(D)   UTILIZATION OF GROUP OR BLANKET HEALTH INSURANCE   215
BENEFITS BY A CERTIFIED NURSE PRACTITIONER IS SUBJECT TO REVIEW   216
BY A PEER REVIEW COMMITTEE APPOINTED BY THE STATE BOARD OF   217
EXAMINERS OF NURSES ~~IN ACCORDANCE WITH THE JOINT REGULATIONS~~   218
~~OF THE BOARD OF MEDICAL EXAMINERS AND THE BOARD OF EXAMINERS~~   219
~~OF NURSES~~.   220
                                                                        221
~~490A-3.~~   222
                                                                        223
~~NOTWITHSTANDING ANY PROVISION OF A GROUP OR INDIVIDUAL~~   224
~~POLICY OR CONTRACT, OR ANY CERTIFICATE ISSUED THEREUNDER, OF~~   225
~~HEALTH, SICKNESS, ACCIDENT, OR DISABILITY INSURANCE THAT IS~~   226
~~WRITTEN ON AN EXPENSE INCURRED BASIS, DELIVERED WITHIN THE~~   227
~~STATE, OR ISSUED TO A GROUP WHICH IS INCORPORATED OR HAS A MAIN~~   228
~~OFFICE LOCATED IN THE STATE, OR COVERING PERSONS WHO RESIDE OR~~   229
~~WORK WITHIN THE STATE, WHENEVER SUCH POLICY, CONTRACT, OR~~   230
~~CERTIFICATE PROVIDES FOR REIMBURSEMENT FOR ANY SERVICE WHICH IS~~   231
~~WITHIN THE LAWFUL SCOPE OF PRACTICE OF A NURSE PRACTITIONER, THE~~   232
~~INSURED, OR ANY OTHER PERSON COVERED BY THE POLICY, CONTRACT,~~   233
~~OR CERTIFICATE, SHALL BE ENTITLED TO REIMBURSEMENT FOR SUCH~~   234
~~SERVICE, WHETHER THE SERVICE IS PERFORMED BY A DOCTOR OF~~   235
~~MEDICINE OR A NURSE PRACTITIONER. THE PROVISIONS OF THIS SECTION~~   236
~~SHALL APPLY TO ALL SUCH POLICIES, CONTRACTS, OR CERTIFICATES~~   237
~~ISSUED, RENEWED, MODIFIED, ALTERED, AMENDED, OR REISSUED ON OR~~   238
~~AFTER JULY 1, 1980.~~   239

House Bill No. 586—*cont'd.*

Continued.

6   HOUSE BILL No. 586

Article 43 - Health   240

241

42.   242

243

     (a) (2) (ii) In this paragraph a "nurse midwife" means a licensed registered   244
nurse who has been certified by the American College of Nurse-Midwives as a nurse   245
midwife AND CERTIFIED NURSE PRACTITIONER MEANS A LICENSED   246
REGISTERED NURSE WHO HAS COMPLETED A NURSE PRACTITIONER   247
PROGRAM APPROVED BY THE STATE BOARD OF EXAMINERS OF NURSES   248
AND PASSED A BOARD APPROVED EXAMINATION~~, AND HAS BEEN~~   249
~~CERTIFIED UNDER THE JOINT REGULATIONS OF THE BOARD OF MEDICAL~~   250
~~EXAMINERS AND THE BOARD OF EXAMINERS OF NURSES~~. For the purposes of   251
this section the nurse midwife need not be under the supervision of a physician. The   252
secretary may contract with nurse midwives or CERTIFIED NURSE   253
PRACTITIONERS for the provision of care for eligible persons. Utilization of benefits   254
under this paragraph by a nurse midwife OR CERTIFIED NURSE PRACTITIONER is   255
subject to a peer review committee appointed by the State Board of Examiners of   256
Nurses ~~IN ACCORDANCE WITH THE JOINT REGULATIONS OF THE BOARD OF~~   257
~~MEDICAL EXAMINERS AND THE BOARD OF EXAMINERS OF NURSES~~.   258

259

294.   260

261

     (a) The Board shall have the following powers and duties: 262

263

        (18) To maintain [an] up-to-date [list] LISTS of all nurse midwives AND   264
CERTIFIED NURSE PRACTITIONERS licensed by the State.   265

266

295.   267

268

     (f) A license issued to any nurse midwife OR CERTIFIED NURSE   269
PRACTITIONER by the Board shall so indicate in an appropriate space on the license.   270

271

301A.   272

273

     (a) (1) In this [section a] SUBSECTION "nurse midwife" means a licensed   274
registered nurse who has been certified by the American College of Nurse-Midwives as   275
a nurse midwife.   276

277

     [(b)] (2) The State Board of Examiners of Nurses shall appoint a peer review   278
committee to provide for oversight of health insurance and medical assistance benefit   279
utilization by nurse midwives.   280

House Bill No. 586—*cont'd.*

Continued.

HOUSE BILL No. 586   7

(B) (1) IN THIS SUBSECTION "CERTIFIED NURSE PRACTITIONER"   281
MEANS A LICENSED REGISTERED NURSE WHO HAS COMPLETED A NURSE   282
PRACTITIONER PROGRAM APPROVED BY THE MARYLAND STATE BOARD OF 283
EXAMINERS OF NURSES AND WHO HAS PASSED A BOARD APPROVED   284
EXAMINATION, AND HAS BEEN CERTIFIED UNDER THE JOINT   285
REGULATIONS OF THE BOARD OF MEDICAL EXAMINERS AND THE BOARD OF 286
EXAMINERS OF NURSES.   287
                                                             288
(2) THE STATE BOARD OF EXAMINERS OF NURSES SHALL APPOINT   289
A PEER REVIEW COMMITTEE TO PROVIDE FOR OVERSIGHT OF HEALTH   290
INSURANCE AND MEDICAL ASSISTANCE BENEFIT UTILIZATION BY   291
CERTIFIED NURSE PRACTITIONERS.   292
                                                             293
SECTION 2. AND BE IT FURTHER ENACTED, That this Act shall take effect   294
January 1, 1980.   295

Approved:

_____

                                   Governor.

_____

                    Speaker of the House of Delegates.

_____

                         President of the Senate.

House Bill No. 586—*cont'd.*

A Daily Synopsis of Bills

Throughout the session each house publishes its own synopsis of bills, which notifies house members of bills and resolutions that have been introduced and the committees to which they have been assigned. Part of a House synopsis is shown on p. 203.*

---

*From the *Student Legislative Handbook,* Maryland General Assembly, Annapolis, Md.

Date Issued   Identification of House or Senate   Synopsis Number

General Assembly of Maryland
Daily Synopsis of Bills & Resolutions
Introduced in The House of Delegates
prepared by the
State Department of Legislative Reference
90 State Circle - Annapolis, Maryland 21401
From Baltimore area - 301/269-3201
Telephone: From Washington, D.C. area - 301/261-2300

DATE ISSUED: February 18, 1980   NUMBER: 24, Page 1

HOUSE OF DELEGATES COMMITTEES			
APPROPRIATIONS	APP	ENVIRONMENTAL MATTERS	ENM
CONSTITUTIONAL AND ADMINISTRATIVE LAW	CAL	JUDICIARY	JUD
ECONOMIC MATTERS	ECM	WAYS AND MEANS	W&M

HB 1949   Hargreaves   CREATION OF A STATE DEBT—RAIL PROPERTY ACQUISITION:
           et al   Authorizing a State Debt of $15,000,000 to be used for
                          rail facilities within and without the State. APP

HB 1950   Neall   RESOURCE RECOVERY AND MATERIALS RECYCLING: Enacting the
           et al   Resource Recovery and Materials Recycling Act; and creat-
                         ing a resource recovery and materials recycling program
                         in the Department of Natural Resources.
                         Md. Ann. Code, Art. 41, Sec. 486(d) amended, and Art. 81,
                         Sec. 468 added, and Natural Resources Article, Sec. 3-701
                         through 3-716 added. ENM and W&M

HB 1951   L Riley   WICOMICO COUNTY—ALCOHOLIC BEVERAGES—BOWLING ALLEYS:
                         Defining the term "bowling alleys" under the Alcoholic
                         Beverages law.
                         Md. Ann. Code, Art. 2B, Sec. 2(w) added. 36th Legislative
                         District, Somerset, Wicomico and Worcester Co.

HB 1952   L Riley   WICOMICO COUNTY—ALCOHOLIC BEVERAGES—HOURS OF SALE:
                         Providing that in Wicomico County the privileges for the
                         sale of certain alcoholic beverages may be exercised at
                         certain hours on a certain day.
                         Md. Ann. Code, Art. 2B, Sec. 84(d) added. 36th Legisla-
                         tive District, Somerset, Wicomico and Worcester Co.

HB 1953   Maloney   STATE LAW ENFORCEMENT EMPLOYEES—OVERTIME COMPENSATION:
           et al   Changing the maximum amount of overtime compensation
                         permitted for certain State law enforcement employees.
                         Md. Ann. Code, Art. 100, Sec. 76(d)(2) amended. APP

HB 1954   Maloney   INSURANCE CODE—SERVICE OF PROCESS: Relating to service
           et al   of process upon insurers as a substitute for service upon
                         a defendant in a motor vehicle tort case.
                         Md. Ann. Code, Art. 48A, Sec. 57A added. ECM

HB 1955   Maloney   CONTROLLED DANGEROUS DRUGS—RULES AND REGULATIONS:
                         Providing that rules and regulations promulgated by the
                         Department of Health and Mental Hygiene and regarding
                         controlled dangerous substances may not place an unneces-
                         sary burden on certain licensed practitioners without a
                         certain showing.
                         Md. Ann. Code, Art. 27, Sec. 280 amended. ENM

Bill Number   Sponsor   Subject Matter   Committee Referred To

Daily Synopsis of Bills & Resolutions Introduced in The House of Delegates.

Committee Report*

Each bill or joint resolution is referred to a committee for study. Members of the committee vote to give the bill or resolution a favorable or unfavorable report. Then they notify the other members of the house by means of a committee report, shown on the next page. This report constitutes the second reading of a bill or resolution.

Twenty-four hour notice is given to the members on bills coming out on the floor for second reading until the last few days of session, when this rule is suspended.

The committee name is always listed at the top and the bills and resolutions are listed from low to high number in their category (favorable or unfavorable). The following will help you understand the information listed on the report.

Distribution Date: Date report is handed out on the floor to members.

Second Reading Date: Date bills and resolutions will be discussed on the floor.

Bill Number: HB = House Bill

                 SB = Senate Bill

                 HJR = House Joint Resolution

                 SJR = Senate Joint Resolution

Report:

     FAV = Favorable as the bill or resolution stands.

     F/A or FAV/A or F/W/A = Favorable, but the committee has amendments to offer.

     NOTE: On the House committee reports you may also see an "s" next to these abbreviations. The House has a screen that it uses to show small amendments. The "s" means that the committee amendments will be shown on the screen instead of being handed out to the members.

     UNF or UNFAV = Unfavorable report by the committee. The bill or resolution usually dies if given this recommendation.

Sponsor: Person(s) who put the bill in for consideration.

Relating To: Brief summary of the bill or resolution.

---

*From the *Student Legislative Handbook,* Maryland General Assembly, Annapolis, Md.

Report of the Committee on **Economic Matters**

| | | DISTRIBUTION DATE | February 1, 1980 |
| | | SECOND READING DATE | February 4, 1980 |

BILL NUMBER	REPORT	SPONSOR	RELATING TO
HB 51	FAV.	McCoy	Baltimore City—Real Estate Practices
HB 482	FAV.	Rummage (Dept.)	Private Detectives—Filing Annual Statement and Renewal Application
HB 496	F/A/S	Pesci	Insurance Code—Exemptions from Provisions
HB 15	UNFAV.	Conaway	Motor Vehicle Installment Sale Agreements—Rebates
HB 67	UNFAV.	Burkhead	Withdrawn by sponsor Alcoholic Beverages—Price Regulation to Include Beer
HB 127	UNFAV.	Garrott	Elevators in Buildings
HB 237	UNFAV.	Maloney et al	Withdrawn by sponsor Alcoholic Beverages—Tax stamps
HB 326	UNFAV.	Hollinger et al	Consumer Goods—Unfair Trade Practices
HB 377	UNFAV.	Pilchard	Worcester Cnty.—Alcoholic Beverages (Ocean City Convention Hall—Purchases) Withdrawn by sponsor
HB 381	UNFAV.	Bienen	Vehicle Laws—Inspection of New Class "A" Vehicles
HB 445	UNFAV.	Garrott	Prepaid Veterinary Care Plans
HB 506	UNFAV.	Winegrad et al	Motor Vehicle Sales—Advertising Fuel Economy
HB 622	UNFAV.	Sprague	Withdrawn by sponsor Employment—Minors Under Fourteen Years of Age

MGA · 11 ·

_____
Chairman

Report of the Committee on Economic Matters.

Third Reading Calendar*

After a bill or joint resolution has passed second reading (the committee report), it is placed on a third reading calendar for final passage.

---

*From the *Student Legislative Handbook,* Maryland General Assembly, Annapolis, Md.

Date Vote Will Be Taken   *Calendar Number*

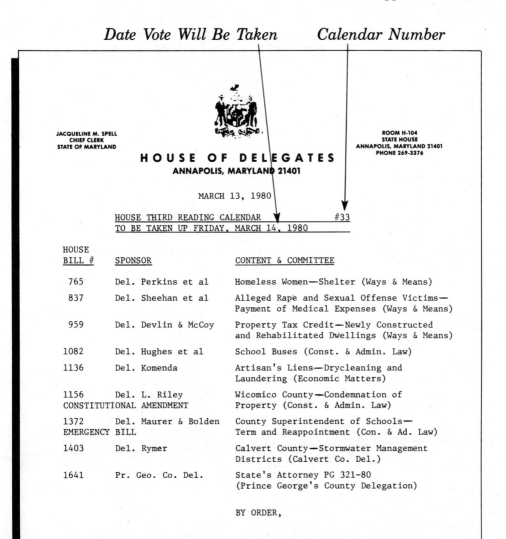

JACQUELINE M. SPELL
CHIEF CLERK
STATE OF MARYLAND

HOUSE OF DELEGATES
ANNAPOLIS, MARYLAND 21401

ROOM H-104
STATE HOUSE
ANNAPOLIS, MARYLAND 21401
PHONE 269-3376

MARCH 13, 1980

HOUSE THIRD READING CALENDAR   #33
TO BE TAKEN UP FRIDAY, MARCH 14, 1980

HOUSE BILL #	SPONSOR	CONTENT & COMMITTEE
765	Del. Perkins et al	Homeless Women—Shelter (Ways & Means)
837	Del. Sheehan et al	Alleged Rape and Sexual Offense Victims—Payment of Medical Expenses (Ways & Means)
959	Del. Devlin & McCoy	Property Tax Credit—Newly Constructed and Rehabilitated Dwellings (Ways & Means)
1082	Del. Hughes et al	School Buses (Const. & Admin. Law)
1136	Del. Komenda	Artisan's Liens—Drycleaning and Laundering (Economic Matters)
1156 CONSTITUTIONAL AMENDMENT	Del. L. Riley	Wicomico County—Condemnation of Property (Const. & Admin. Law)
1372 EMERGENCY BILL	Del. Maurer & Bolden	County Superintendent of Schools—Term and Reappointment (Con. & Ad. Law)
1403	Del. Rymer	Calvert County—Stormwater Management Districts (Calvert Co. Del.)
1641	Pr. Geo. Co. Del.	State's Attorney PG 321-80 (Prince George's County Delegation)

BY ORDER,

JACQUELINE M. SPELL
CHIEF CLERK

Third Reading Calendar.

MARYLAND GENERAL ASSEMBLY
DEPARTMENT OF FISCAL SERVICES
DIVISION OF FISCAL RESEARCH
JOSEPH M. COBLE, DIRECTOR

FISCAL NOTE

SB 651

Senate Bill 651 (Senator Hollinger, et al)

Economic and Environmental Affairs

SUMMARY OF LEGISLATION: In defining "area of shortage" to mean the average statewide employment vacancy rate of licensed health occupations at hospitals or related institutions exceeds 7%, this bill requires the Secretary of Health and Mental Hygiene to undertake annually: (1) a survey of hospitals and institutions for areas of shortage, and (2) make 5-year projections on the average statewide areas of shortage and the number of students expected to graduate and become licensed in those areas of shortage.

All boards and commissions in the Health-Occupations Article are to provide the Secretary with the information the Secretary needs for these activities. Each year, the Secretary is required to report the results of this annual survey to the General Assembly, the Governor, the State Board for Higher Education, and the State Board for Community Colleges.

STATE FISCAL IMPACT STATEMENT: Excluding the $50,000 budgeted for the Nurse Database now being programmed, the Department of Health and Mental Hygiene estimates that additional expenditures of $60,000 to $100,000 annually will be required to implement this bill.

The Department of Fiscal Services believes that these costs can be reduced in future years, as illustrated below. State revenues are not affected.

LOCAL FISCAL IMPACT STATEMENT: No effect.

STATE REVENUES: No effect.

STATE EXPENDITURES: The Department of Health and Mental Hygiene reports that it has to ascertain the information currently available before it can determine a need for additional resources to comply with the provisions of this bill. The Nurse Database being programmed for its annual renewal system can be used by all the health occupation boards. The Department estimates that $50,000 in additional expenditures will be required to collect the data required by this bill, which includes printing and postage.

Another $10,000 is estimated to survey all hospitals and related institutions, using data systems under development.

Continued.

The cost to survey schools, colleges, and universities is not known. The Department of Fiscal Services believes that educational institutions can focus on the number of health occupation candidates graduating annually, from which reliable estimates can be developed for the number who will become licensed. A correlation will be required between areas of shortage in hospitals and related institutions throughout the State and licensed graduates. Trade associations such as the Maryland Hospital Association and the Health Facilities Association of Maryland should be helpful in this respect.

The Department of Health and Mental Hygiene feels that it will be unable to absorb within existing resources the overall data analysis, projections, and preparation of the annual survey.

The Department of Fiscal Services estimates additional expenditures as shown below.

LOCAL REVENUES: No effect.

LOCAL EXPENDITURES: No effect.

State Impact	FY 1989	FY 1990	FY 1991	FY 1992	FY 1993
Revenues	0	0	0	0	0
Expenditures	$78,000	$46,300	$37,300	$28,300	$29,300
Net Effect	($78,000)	($46,300)	($37,300)	($28,300)	($29,300)

( ) Indicates Decrease

INFORMATION SOURCE: DHMH

ESTIMATE BY: DFS

Fiscal Note History: First Reader - February 29, 1988

Per: E.P. Sayre   John Lang, III, Supervising Analyst
      nlr   Division of Fiscal Research

Senate Bill 651
Page Two

APPENDIX E: NAMES, ADDRESSES, AND TELEPHONE NUMBERS OF NURSING ORGANIZATIONS

American Nurses' Association
2420 Pershing Rd
Kansas City, MO 64108

Advocates for Child Psychiatric Nursing
603 Shakertown Ct
Cincinnati, OH 45242

American Academy of Ambulatory
  Nursing Administration
North Woodbury Rd
PO Box 56
Pitman, NJ 08071

American Academy of Nurse Practitioners
893 Stone Jug Rd
Biglerville, PA 17307

American Assembly for Men in Nursing
PO Box 31753
Independence, OH 44131

American Association of Colleges of
  Nursing
1 Dupont Circle, NW
Suite 530
Washington, DC 20036

American Association of Critical Care
  Nurses
1 Civic Plaza
Newport Beach, CA 92660

American Association of Diabetes
  Educators
500 N Michigan Avenue
#1400
Chicago, IL 60611

American Association of Neuroscience
  Nurses
218 N Jefferson
Suite 204
Chicago, IL 60606

American Association of Nurse
  Anesthetists
216 Higgins Rd
Park Ridge, IL 60068

American Association of Nurse Attorneys
113 W Franklin St
Baltimore, MD 21201

American Association of Nursing History
1753 W Congress Plaza
Chicago, IL 60612

American Association of Occupational
  Health Nurses
50 Lenox Pointe
Atlanta, GA 30324

American Association of Spinal Cord
  Injury Nurses
432 Park Ave S
New York, NY 10016

American College of Nurse Midwives
1522 K St NW
Suite 1000
Washington, DC 20005

American Holistic Nurses' Association
Rt 4, PO Box 365B
Carbondale, IL 62901

American Nephrology Nurses' Association
N Woodbury Rd
PO Box 56
Pitman, NJ 08071

American Organization of Nurse
  Executives
840 N Lake Shore Dr
Chicago, IL 60611

American Psychiatric Nurses Association
c/o Shirley Smoyak
Rutgers College of Nursing
4 Roney Rd
Edison, NJ 08820

American Public Health Association,
  Public Health Nurses
1015 15th St NW
Washington, DC 20005

This list was provided courtesy of the Nurses' Association of the American College of Obstetrics and Gynecology. An updated directory is published annually in the April issue of the American Journal of Nursing.

American Society for Parental & Enteral
Nutrition, Nurses Committee
8605 Cameron St
Suite 500
Silver Spring, MD 20910

American Society of Ophthalmic
Registered Nurses, Inc
655 Beach St
PO Box 3030
San Francisco, CA 94119

American Society of Plastic &
Reconstructive Surgical Nurses
N Woodbury Rd
PO Box 56
Pitman, NJ 08071

American Society of Post Anesthesia
Nurses
11508 Allecingie Parkway
Suite C
Richmond, VA 23235

American Urological Association Allied
Shore Dr
PO Box 9397
Raytown, MO 64133

Arthritis Health Professionals
Association, Nursing Section
Columbia Hospital
2025 E Newport
Milwaukee, WI 53211

Association for Practitioners in Infection
Control
505 E Hawley
Mundelein, IL 60060

Association of Faculties of Pediatric
Nurse Practitioners and Associates
Programs
c/o Linda Gilman
5250 N Meridian
Indianapolis, IN 46208

Association of Operating Room Nurses
10170 E Mississippi Ave
Denver, CO 80231

Association of Pediatric Oncology Nurses
6728 Old McLean Village
McLean, VA 22101

Association of Rehabilitation Nurses
2506 Gross Point Rd
Evanston, IL 60201

Chi Eta Phi Sorority, Inc.
2247 Glendale Dr
Decatur, GA 30032

Commission of Graduates of Foreign
Nursing Schools
3624 Mailut
Philadelphia, PA 19104

Consortium of Registered Nurses for Eye
Acquisition
1511 K St NW
Suite 830
Washington, DC 20005

Dermatology Nurses Association
N Woodbury Rd
PO Box 56
Pitman, NJ 08071

Drug and Alcohol Nursing Association
113 W Franklin St
Baltimore, MD 21201

Emergency Nurses Association
230 E Ohio
Suite 600
Chicago, IL 60611

International Association for
Enterostomal Therapy
2081 Business Center Ct
#290
Irvine, CA 92715

Intravenous Nurses Society
2 Brighten St
Belmont, MA 02178

NAACOG
409 12th St SW
Washington, DC 20024-2191

National Alliance of Nurse Practitioners
PO Box 44707
L'Enfant Plaza SW
Washington, DC 20026

National Association for Health Care
Recruitment
PO Box 93851
Cleveland, OH 44101-5851

National Association of Hispanic Nurses
2014 Johnston St
Los Angeles, CA 90031

National Association of Neonatal Nurses
177 Lynch Creek Way
Petaluma, CA 94952

National Association of Nurse
Practitioners in Family Planning
810 7th Ave 7th Floor
New York, NY 10019

National Association of Orthopaedic
Nurses
N Woodbury Rd
PO Box 56
Pitman, NJ 08071

National Association of Pediatric Nurse
Associates & Practitioners
1101 Kings Highway N
Suite 206
Cherry Hill, NJ 08034

National Association of School Nurses,
Inc
Lamplighter Lane
PO Box 1300
Scarborough, ME 04074

National Black Nurses Association, Inc
1011 N Capitol St NE
Washington, DC 20002

National Conference of Gerontological
Nurse Practitioners
c/o Linda Grissom
Institute for Human Services
3501 N Scottsdale Rd
#320
Scottsdale, AZ 85251

National Council of State Board of
Nursing
625 N Michigan Ave
Suite 1544
Chicago, IL 60611

National Federation of Specialty Nursing
Organizations
L'Enfant Plaza SW
PO Box 23836
Washington, DC 20026

National Flight Nurses Association
PO Box 8222
Rapid City, SD 57709

National Gerontological Nursing
Association
6621 Adrian St
New Carrollton, MD 20784

National League for Nursing
10 Columbus Circle
New York, NY 10019

National Nurses in Business Association
4286 Redwood Highway
Suite 252
San Rafael, CA 94903

National Nurses Society on Addictions
2506 Gross Point Rd
Evanston, IL 60201

National Organization for Nurse
Practitioners Faculties
NP Program, Himmelfarb Library
2300 Eye St NW
Washington, DC 20037

National Organization for Philippine
Nurses in US
459 Joan St
South Plainfield, NJ 07080

National Student Nurses Association
555 W 57th St
Room 1325
New York, NY 10019

North American Nursing Diagnosis
Association
c/o St Louis University
School of Nursing
3525 Caroline St
St. Louis, MO 63104

Nurse Consultants Association
414 Plaza Dr
Suite 209
Westmont, IL 60559

Nurses' Environmental Health Watch
2110 Fourth St
Suite 26
Santa Monica, CA 90405

Nurses Organization of the Veterans
Administration
6728 Old McLean Village
McLean, VA 22101

Oncology Nursing Society
1016 Greentree Rd
Pittsburgh, PA 15220

Pediatric Endocrinology Nursing Society
2545 Chicago Ave S
Suite 408
Minneapolis, MN 55404

Sigma Theta Tau
1100 Waterway Blvd
Indianapolis, IN 46202

Society for Education & Research in Psyc/
  MH Nursing
c/o Ann Cain, PhD
1106 Little Magothy View
Cape St Clair
Annapolis, MD 21401

Society for Peripheral Vascular Nursing
1070 Sibley Tower
Rochester, NY 14604

Society of Gastrointestinal Assistants
1070 Sibley Tower
Rochester, NY 14604

Society of Otorhinolaryngology & Head-
  Neck Nurses, Inc.
4330 Sea Mist Dr
New Smyrna Beach, FL 32069

The Association of Nurses in AIDS Care
CN5254
Princeton, NJ 08543-5254

The Society of Nursing History
Nursing Education Department
Box 150
Teachers College
Columbia University
New York, NY 10027

Transcultural Nursing Society
College of Nursing
University of Utah
25 S Dr
Salt Lake City, UT 84112

State and Territorial Nurses' Associations

Asterisk (*) denotes SNAs that have political action committees (PACs).

Alabama*
Alabama State Nurses' Association
360 N Hull St
Montgomery, AL 36197
(205) 262-8321

Alaska*
Alaska Nurses Association
237 E Third Ave
Anchorage, AK 99501
(907) 274-0827 or (907) 264-1706

Arizona*
Arizona Nurses' Association
Suite 1
1850 E Southern Ave
Tempe, AZ 85282
(602) 831-0404

Arkansas*
Arkansas State Nurses' Association
117 S Cedar St
Little Rock, AR 72205
(501) 664-5853

California*
California Nurses Association
1855 Folsom St
Room 670
San Francisco, CA 94103
(415) 864-4141

Colorado*
Colorado Nurses' Association
5453 E Evans Place
Denver, CO 80222
(303) 757-7484

Connecticut*
Connecticut Nurses' Association
Meritech Business Park
377 Research Parkway
Suite 2D
Meriden, CT 06450
(203) 238-1207

Delaware*
Delaware Nurses' Association
2634 Capitol Trail
Suite C
Newark, DE 19711
(302) 368-2333

This list was provided courtesy of the American Nurses' Association.

District of Columbia*
District of Columbia Nurses' Association,
  Inc
5100 Wisconsin Ave NW
Suite 306
Washington, DC 20016
(202) 244-2705

Florida*
Florida Nurses Association
1235 E Concord St
PO Box 536985
Orlando, FL 32853
(407) 896-3261

Georgia*
Georgia Nurses Association, Inc.
1362 W Peachtree St NW
Atlanta, GA 30309
(404) 876-4624

Hawaii*
Hawaii Nurses' Association
677 Ala Moana Blvd
Suite 601
Honolulu, HI 96813
(808) 531-1628

Idaho*
Idaho Nurses Association
200 N Fourth St
Suite 20
Boise, ID 83702-6001
(208) 345-0500

Illinois*
Illinois Nurses Association
20 N Wacker Dr
Suite 2520
Chicago, IL 60606
(312) 236-9708

Indiana
Indiana State Nurses' Associaton
2915 N High School Rd
Indianapolis, IN 46224
(317) 299-4575 or 4576

Iowa*
Iowa Nurses' Association
100 Court Ave, 9LL
Des Moines, IA 50309
(515) 282-9169

Kansas
Kansas State Nurses Association
820 Quincy St
Topeka, KS 66612
(913) 233-8638

Kentucky*
Kentucky Nurses Association
1400 S First St
PO Box 2616
Louisville, KY 40201
(502) 637-2546 or 2547

Louisiana*
Lousiana State Nurses Association
712 Transcontinental Dr
Metairie, LA 70001
(504) 889-1030

Maine
Maine State Nurses' Association
PO Box 2240
Augusta, ME 04330
(207) 622-1057

Maryland*
Maryland Nurses Association, Inc.
5820 Southwestern Blvd
Baltimore, MD 21227
(301) 242-7300

Massachusetts*
Massachusetts Nurses' Association
340 Turnpike St
Canton, MA 02021
(617) 821-4625

Michigan*
Michigan Nurses Association
120 Spartan Ave
East Lansing, MI 48823
(517) 337-1653

Minnesota*
Minnesota Nurses Association
1295 Bandana Blvd N
Suite 140
St. Paul, MN 55108
(612) 646-4807

Mississippi*
Mississippi Nurses' Association
135 Bounds St
Suite 100
Jackson, MS 39206
(601) 982-9182 or 9183

Missouri*
Missouri Nurses Association
206 East Dunklin St
PO Box 325
Jefferson City, MO 65101
(314) 636-4623

Montana*
Montana Nurses' Association
715 Getchell
PO Box 5718
Helena, MT 59604
(406) 442-6710

Nebraska*
Nebraska Nurses' Association
941 'O' St
Suite 707-711
Lincoln, NE 68508
(402) 475-3859

Nevada*
Nevada Nurses' Association
3660 Baker Lane
Suite 104
Reno, NV 89509
(702) 825-3555

New Hampshire*
New Hampshire Nurses' Association
48 West St
Concord, NH 03301
(603) 225-3783

New Jersey*
New Jersey State Nurses Association
320 W State St
Trenton, NJ 08618
(609) 392-4884 or 2031

New Mexico*
New Mexico Nurses' Association
525 San Pedro, NE
Suite 100
Albuquerque, NM 87108
(505) 268-7744

New York*
New York State Nurses Association
2113 Western Ave
Guilderland, NY 12084
(518) 456-5371

North Carolina*
North Carolina Nurses Association
103 Enterprise St
PO Box 12025
Raleigh, NC 27605
(919) 821-4250

North Dakota*
North Dakota Nurses' Association
Green Tree Square
212 N Fourth St
Bismarck, ND 58501
(701) 223-1385

Ohio*
Ohio Nurses Association
4000 E Main St
Columbus, OH 43213-2950
(614) 237-5414

Oklahoma*
Oklahoma Nurses Association
6414 N Santa Fe
Suite A
Oklahoma City, OK 73116
(405) 840-3476

Oregon*
Oregon Nurses Association, Inc.
9700 SW Capitol Highway
Suite 200
Portland, OR 97219
(503) 293-0011

Pennsylvania*
Pennsylvania Nurses Association
2578 Interstate Dr
PO Box 8525
Harrisburg, PA 17105-8525
(717) 657-1222

Rhode Island
Rhode Island State Nurses' Association
Hall Building South
345 Blackstone Blvd
Providence, RI 02906
(401) 421-9703

South Carolina*
South Carolina Nurses' Association
1821 Gadsden St
Columbia, SC 29201
(803) 252-4781

South Dakota*
South Dakota Nurses' Association, Inc.
1505 S Minnesota
Suite 6
Sioux Falls, SD 57105
(605) 338-1401

Tennessee*
Tennessee Nurses' Association
1720 West End Building
Suite 400
Nashville, TN 37203
(615) 329-2511

Texas*
Texas Nurses Association
Community Bank Building
300 Highland Mall Blvd
Suite 300
Austin, TX 78752-3718
(512) 452-0645

Utah*
Utah Nurses' Association
1058A E 900 S
Salt Lake City, UT 84105
(801) 322-3439 or 3430

Vermont
Vermont State Nurses' Association, Inc.
500 Dorset St
South Burlington, VT 05403
(802) 864-9390

Virginia*
Virginia Nurses' Association
1311 High Point Ave
Richmond, VA 23230
(804) 353-7311

Washington*
Washington State Nurses Association
83 S King St
Suite 500
Seattle, WA 98104
(206) 622-3613

West Virginia*
West Virginia Nurses Association, Inc.
2 Players Club Dr
Building 3
PO Box 1946
Charleston, WV 25327
(304) 342-1169

Wisconsin*
Wisconsin Nurses Association, Inc.
6117 Monona Dr
Madison, WI 53716
(608) 221-0383

Wyoming
Wyoming Nurses Association
Majestic Building
Room 305
1603 Capitol Avenue
Cheyenne, WY 82001
(307) 635-3955

Guam
Guam Nurses' Association
PO Box 3134
Agana, GU 96910
(671) 646-5801 or 6711

Virgin Islands
Virgin Islands Nurses' Association
PO Box 583
Christiansted
St. Croix, VI 00820
(809) 773-2323, Ext. 116 or 118

The National Council of State Boards of Nursing, Member Boards

Alabama
Alabama Board of Nursing
500 Eastern Blvd
Suite 203
Montgomery, AL 36117
(205) 261-4060

Alaska
Alaska Board of Nursing
Department of Commerce and Economic
    Development
Division of Occupational Licensing
3601 C Street
Suite 722
Anchorage, AK 99503
(907) 561-2878

This list was provided courtesy of the Maryland Board of Nursing.

Arizona
Arizona State Board of Nursing
2001 W Camelback Rd
Suite 350
Phoenix, AZ 85015
(602) 255-5092

Arkansas
Arkansas State Board of Nursing
1123 S University
Little Rock, AR 72204
(501) 371-2751

California
California Board of Registered Nursing
PO Box 944210
Sacramento, CA 94244-2100
(916) 322-3350

California Board of Vocational Nurse and
Psychiatric Technician Examiners
1414 K St
Sacramento, CA 95814
(916) 445-0793

Colorado
Colorado Board of Nursing
1560 Broadway
Suite 670
Denver, CO 80202
(303) 894-2430

Connecticut
Connecticut Board of Examiners for
Nursing
150 Washington St
Hartford, CT 06106
(203) 566-1041

Delaware
Delaware Board of Nursing
Margaret O'Neill Building
PO Box 1401
Dover, DE 19901
(302) 736-4522

District of Columbia
District of Columbia Board of Nursing
614 H. Street NW
Washington, DC 20001
(202) 727-7468

Florida
Florida Board of Nursing
111 Coastline Dr E
Jacksonville, FL 32202
(904) 359-6331

Georgia
Georgia Board of Nursing
166 Pryor St SW
Atlanta, GA 30303
(404) 656-3943

Georgia State Board of Licensed Practical
Nurses
166 Pryor St SW
Atlanta, GA 30303
(404) 656-3921

Hawaii
Hawaii Board of Nursing
PO Box 3469
Honolulu, HI 96801
(808) 548-3086

Idaho
Idaho Board of Nursing
500 S 10th St
Suite 102
Boise, ID 83720
(208) 334-3110

Illinois
Illinois Department of Professional
Regulation
320 W Washington St
Springfield, IL 62786
(217) 785-0800

Indiana
Indiana State Board of Nursing
Health Professions Bureau
1 American Square
Suite 1020
Box 82067
Indianapolis, IN 46282-0004
(317) 232-2960

Iowa
Iowa Board of Nursing
Executive Hills East
1223 East Ct
Des Moines, IA 50319
(515) 281-3256

Kansas
Kansas Board of Nursing
Landon State Office Building
900 SW Jackson
Suite 551 S
Topeka, KS 66612-1256
(913) 296-4929

Kentucky
Kentucky Board of Nursing
4010 Dupont Circle
Suite 430
Louisville, KY 40207
(502) 897-5143

Louisiana
Louisiana State Board of Nursing
907 Pere Marquette Building
150 Baronne St
New Orleans, LA 70112
(504) 568-5464

Louisiana State Board of Practical Nurse
  Examiners
Tidewater Place
1440 Canal St
Suite 2010
New Orleans, LA 70112
(504) 568-6480

Maine
Maine State Board of Nursing
295 Water St
Augusta, ME 04330
(207) 289-5324

Maryland
Maryland Board of Examiners of Nurses
4201 Patterson Ave
Baltimore, MD 21215-2299
(301) 764-4747 or 2480

Massachusetts
Massachusetts Board of Registration in
  Nursing
Leverett Saltonstall Building
100 Cambridge St
Room 1519
Boston, MA 02202
(617) 727-7393

Michigan
Michigan Board of Nursing
Department of Licensing and Regulation
Ottawa Towers North
611 W Ottawa
PO Box 30018
Lansing, MI 48909
(517) 373-1600

Minnesota
Minnesota Board of Nursing
2700 University Ave W, #108
St. Paul, MN 55114
(612) 642-0567

Mississippi
Mississippi Board of Nursing
239 N Lamar St
Suite 401
Jackson, MS 39206-1311
(601) 359-6170

Missouri
Missouri State Board of Nursing
PO Box 656
3523 N Ten Mile Dr
Jefferson City, MO 65102
(314) 751-2334, Ext. 141

Montana
Montana State Board of Nursing
Department of Commerce, Division of
  Business and Professional Licensing
1424 Ninth Ave
Helena, MT 59620-0407
(406) 444-4279

Nebraska
Bureau of Examining Boards
Nebraska Department of Health
PO Box 95007
Lincoln, NE 68509
(402) 471-2115 or 4358

Nevada
Nevada State Board of Nursing
1281 Terminal Way
Suite 116
Reno, NV 89502
(702) 786-2778

New Hampshire
New Hampshire Board of Nursing
Health and Welfare Building
6 Hazen Dr
Concord, NH 03301
(603) 271-2323

New Jersey
New Jersey Board of Nursing
1100 Raymond Blvd
Room 508
Newark, NJ 07102
(201) 648-2570

New Mexico
New Mexico Board of Nursing
4253 Montgomery Blvd
Suite 130
Albuquerque, NM 87109
(505) 841-8340

New York
New York State Board for Nursing
State Education Department
Cultural Education Center
Room 3013
Albany, NY 12230
(518) 474-3843 or 3845

North Carolina
North Carolina Board of Nursing
PO Box 2129
Raleigh, NC 27602
(919) 782-3211

North Dakota
North Dakota Board of Nursing
919 S Seventh St
Suite 504
Bismarck, ND 58504
(701) 224-2974

Ohio
Ohio Board of Nursing Education and
   Nurse Registration
77 S High St
Seventeenth Floor
Columbus, OH 43266-0316
(614) 466-3947

Oklahoma
Oklahoma Board of Nurse Registration
   and Nursing Education
2915 North Classen Blvd
Suite 524
Oklahoma City, OK 73106
(405) 525-2076

Oregon
Oregon State Board of Nursing
1400 SW Fifth Ave
Room 904
Portland, OR 97201
(503) 229-5653

Pennsylvania
Pennsylvania Board of Nursing
Department of State
PO Box 2649
Harrisburg, PA 17105
(717) 787-8503

Rhode Island
Rhode Island Board of Nurse
   Registration and Nursing Education
Cannon Health Building
75 Davis St
Room 104
Providence, RI 02908-2488
(401) 277-2827

South Carolina
South Carolina State Board of Nursing
1777 St Julian Place
Suite 102
Columbia, SC 29204-2488
(803) 737-6594

South Dakota
South Dakota Board of Nursing
304 S Phillips Ave
Suite 205
Sioux Falls, SD 57102
(605) 335-4973

Tennessee
Tennessee State Board of Nursing
283 Plus Park Blvd
Nashville, TN 37217
(615) 367-6232

Texas
Texas Board of Nurse Examiners
PO Box 140466
Austin, TX 78714
(512) 835-4880

Texas Board of Vocational Nurse
   Examiners
PO Box 141007
Austin, TX 78714-1007
(512) 835-2071

Utah
Utah State Board of Nursing
Division of Occupational and Professional
   Licensing
Heber M. Wells Building, Fourth Floor
160 E 300 S
PO Box 45802
Salt Lake City, UT 84145
(801) 530-6628

Vermont
Vermont State Board of Nursing
Redstone Building
26 Terrace St
Montpelier, VT 05602
(802) 828-2396

Virginia
Virginia State Board of Nursing
1601 Rolling Hills Dr
Richmond, VA 23229-5005
(804) 662-9909

Washington
Washington State Board of Nursing
Department of Licensing
PO Box 9649
Olympia, WA 98504
(206) 753-2206

Washington State Board of Practical
  Nursing
PO Box 9012
Olympia, WA 98504
(206) 753-2807

West Virginia
West Virginia Board of Examiners for
  Registered Nurses
922 Quarrier St
Embleton Building
Suite 309
Charleston, WV 25301
(304) 348-3596

West Virginia State Board of Examiners
  for Practical Nurses
922 Quarrier St
Embleton Building
Suite 506
Charleston, WV 25301
(304) 348-3572

Wisconsin
Wisconsin Bureau of Health Professions
1400 E Washington Ave
PO Box 8935
Madison, WI 53708-8935
(608) 266-3735

Wyoming
Wyoming State Board of Nursing
Barrett Building, Fourth Floor
2301 Central Ave
Cheyenne, WY 82002
(307) 777-7601

American Samoa
American Samoa Health Service
  Regulatory Board
LBJ Tropical Medical Center
Pago Pago, American Samoa 96799
(684) 633-1222, Ext. 206
Telex No.: #782-573-LBJ TMC

Guam
Guam Board of Nurse Examiners
PO Box 2816
Agana, GU 96910
0-11-671-734-5500
FAX No.: 0-11-671-734-5910

Northern Mariana Islands
Commonwealth Board of Nurse
  Examiners
Public Health Center
PO Box 1458
Saipan, MP 96950
0-11-670-234-8950, 8951, 8952, 8953, or
  8954
Ask for Public Health Center, Ext. 2018
  or 2019.
Telex No.: 783-744. Answer back code:
  PNESPN744.

Virgin Islands
Virgin Islands Board of Nursing
Knud Hansen Complex
Charlotte Amalie
St. Thomas, VI 00801
(809) 776-7397

Another Reference—*The American Journal of Nursing*'s "Directory of Nursing Organizations"

Each year in its April issue, *The American Journal of Nursing* publishes a complete, up-to-date "Directory of Nursing Organizations." In addition to the information contained in this appendix, the *AJN* Directory includes names, addresses, telephone numbers, and in some cases contact persons in international organizations; a more complete list of national nursing organizations and other organizations that have nursing departments; the ANA's offices and departments; and nursing departments within the U.S. government, including the military and public health services.

APPENDIX F: TIPS FOR PAC FUNDRAISING

- Be sure you understand the laws in your state pertaining to PACs.
- Fundraising literature should briefly explain how the money will be used.
- Make appeals for money personally—people respond more generously to personal appeals.
- Follow up with "thank you" notes. They encourage more giving.
- Keep a list of donors. Frequently they will give again.
- Raffles, bake sales, and 50/50 drawings are simple to organize, and they bring in money. They can be held at almost any nurses' gathering.
- Sales of SNA/PAC buttons are money-makers.
- Fund-raisers featuring a political speaker (especially a PAC-endorsed candidate) are effective. But the event must be well publicized.

INDEX